Assess Recombinant DNA
of
Toxicology

Dr. Jagjeet Singh

Mahaveer & Sons
(Publishers & Distributors)
New Delhi–110002

Edition 2015

ISBN-81-8377-023-1

Published by
MAHAVEER & SONS
3072/28, First Floor, Gola Market, Darya Ganj,
New Delhi–110002

Rs. 750/-

PRINTED IN INDIA

Published by Sh. Mukul Sharma for Mahaveer & Sons, 3072/28, First Floor, Gola Market, Darya Ganj, New Delhi–110002, Printed at Nav Prabhat Printing Press, Delhi.

Preface

This book is the scientific and analytical study of 'Asses Recombinant DNA of Toxicology' Toxicology plays a vital role in the medicolegal investigation of death, whether by alcohol, poison, drugs or any other causes. In the beginning chapter the foundation, of Toxicology and its components and the important roles of Forensic Laboratory and Forensic Toxicologist have been discussed in detail. In the second chapter the fours falls upon relationship between Epidemiology and Toxicology : "Epidemiology and toxicology differ in other ways but principally in that epidemiology is essentially an observational science, in contrast to the experimental method of toxicology." Different type say toxicology–Pharmaceutical Toxicology Neurotoxicology, Combustion Toxicology, Toxicology of the Adrenal, Thyroid and Endocrine Pancreas, Radiation Toxicology are analyse in subsequent chapters.

In the third chapter Pharmaceutical Toxicology to control the drug disaster and pecantions to reduce the death, caused by drug-epidemics are stressed. In attempting to ensure the safety of drugs the licensing Authority and the committee on safety of Medicines in the UK very on three strategies—the control of quality, rigorous pre-marketing safety studies and post-marketing surveillance. Quality is controlled in relation to both manufacture and wholesale selling and, as a consequence, toxicity due to product defects in now exceptional. r-DNA is defined as "either molecules which are constructed outside living cells by joining natural or synthetic DNA segmente of DNA molecules that can replicate in a living cell or DNA molecules the result from their replication—in the next chapter. Fifth chapter dears with the responses of the kidney to toxic compounds. The toxic effect the kidney some or of all its function such as blood urea nitrogen, or creatinine, and the presence of glucose, protein or electrotypes in urine in which are commonly monitored as indicators of renal dys function.

In Poisons of Animal Origin, the vast number of poisonous and venomous animals as well as significant differences among these species, prohibits generations are reviewed. Snakes are categorised by the primary toxic effects of their venom. Snake venom is as complex mixture of protein, enzymes, metals and other inorganic substances. Toxic manifestation, symptoms and management of snakes, Gila monster, Hymenoptera, Ant, spider, Black widow spider, Necrotic, Arachnidism, Scorpions, Jelly fish, stingrays, Poisonous fish have been focused. Further in the same chapter different types of poisonous fish and different cause of toxic manifestation and management have been summarized in brief. In tenth chapter entitled Radiation Toxicology, the effects of Non-stochastic & Radiation toxic on the skin, The Reproductive system, the Digestive System, The Respiratory System, The Nervous System, The Cardiovascular system, The Endocrine system, The Urinary Tract, The Musculaskeletal system have been described.

The concluding chapter is involved with the plannings to prevent disasters. This is followed by an evaluation of different types of disalters or serious incident involving toxicants. Although purely environmental effect should not be ignored, the examples chosen are all associates with human health effects. Afterwards approaches to the planning associated with preventing disasters due to toxicants are mitigating their effects are discussed.

—Editor

Contents

1

Forensic Toxicology

The Toxicology Process

Toxicology plays an important part in the medicolegal investigation of death. It answers the question of whether alcohol, other drugs and or chemical poisons were the cause or a contributory cause of the death. The laboratory can analyse biological specimens including blood, urine, vitreous, bile, tissues (liver, brain, kidney, spleen) and non-biologicals such as pills, air samples and clothing for many toxicants.

Once the laboratory has determined the absence or presence of a drug or chemical toxicant, the toxicologist will give an opinion as to whether the findings are significant and how they may have been related to the death. As drug effects may differ from individual to individual and depend on many factors [health status of an individual, age, sex, combination of drugs detected, quantity of drug taken, manner of dosing (oral, inhalation, injection) and rate of consumption], interpretation is a difficult and complex task based on knowledge and experience.

Foundations of Toxicology

Knowledge about poisons existed as long ago as the ancient writings of the Egyptains which made reference to poisons from plants. A passage from an ancient papyrus has been translated as 'Speak not of the name of Yao under penalty of the peach', indicating knowledge of a poison (hydrocaynic acid) in parts of the peach tree or fruit (Gettler, 1956). The papyrus Ebers from 1500 BC also mentions antimony, copper, hyoscyamus, lead and opium as poisons. Writings from India during the period 600 to 100 BC metion poisons including gold, copper, iron, lead, silver and tin. Socrates was exectued in 339 BC with an extract of hemlock. A book entitled *The History of Plants* published in 300 BC by Theophrastus refers to medicinal and poisonous plants.

Numerous poisonings have been recorded in the history of the first 1800 years after Christ. Nine of the successors of Charlemagne (Holy Roman Empire) died before the 1400s of poisonings. Famous poisonings included five popoes many cardinals, and several kings. It became commonplace for kings to have 'tasters' of their food. In 1552 Nux Vomica (strychnine) was described.

Many poisonings occurred in England, France and Italy during the 16th and 17th Centuries. Spara in the 1650s was the leader of a secret poisoning society in Rome. In the 1700s Madame Toffana of Naples poisoned over 600 victims with white arsenic. The poisons most frequently used in this period were hemlock, aconite, opium, arsenic and corrosive sublimate (mercury).

Up until the late 1700s convictions of perpetrators of homicidal poisonings were based on circumstantial evidence. In 1781, Joseph Plenic stated that the detection and identification of the poison in the organs of the deceased was the only true sign of poisoning.

Matheiw J. B. Orfila (1787–1853) was a Spanish chemist who became a professor of lega medicine at the University of Paris. He published the first complete work international importance on the subject of poisons and legal medicine in 1813. The publication was entitled: *Traite des Poisons Tires des Regnes Mineral Vegetal et Animal, ou Toxicologie Generale.* Orfila is ocnsidered the 'Father of Toxicology'. He identified several different disciplines of toxicology including pharmaceutical, clinical, industrial and environmental. He established many of the guiding principles of toxicology including the need for adequate proof of identity and quality assurances. These principles still true today. They are:

(1) Expericen is paramount for credibility and reliability.
(2) All facts surrounding the case must be given to the analysts.
(3) All the evidence must be submitted properly identified and labelled and sealed.
(4) All tests should be run and properly recorded.
(5) Reagents must be pure, blank tests must be run.
(6) All tests should be repeated and compared to spiked knowns.

Devising analytical methods for the determination of poisons in human organs was one of Orfila's most important accomplishments. In 1839, Orfilla extracted arsenic from human tissues using a procedure for identification developed several years before by James Marsch. This evidence was used in court (1840) to convict Marie Lafarge of a homicidal poisoning. This was the first time toxicological data had been used as evidence in a trial. He was also the instructor of Robert Christions (1779–1882), a British physician who returned to Great Britain after his education. Christison became a professor of legal medicine at the University of Edinburgh and is considered the first British toxicologist. In 1829, he wrote the text *Treatise on Poisons* which was introduced into the USA in 1845.

Some of the major events that led to the development of chemical toxicological (Gettler, 1956), were:

* In 1836, the development of a test for arsenic by James M. Marsh.
* In 1839, Orfilla successfully applied the Marsh test to identify arsenic extracted from liver, kidneys, spleen, muscle and heart.
* In 1844, Freenius and von Babo developed a procedure for the systematic search for all mineral poisons. The procedure used wet ashing with chlorine.
* In 1850, Stas developed a procedure for the extraction of nicotine from human tissues. The method was

modified in 1856 by Otto to give purer extract of alkaloids. This modified procedure is commonly called the Stas–Otto Method.

* In 1874, Salami proved that decomposition can create artefacts and that extreme caution must be used in identification of poisons after death.

During the period from the 1830s the early 1900s, analysis of tissue from human organs for toxicans still remained textremely rare. Most analyses were performed on gastric contents. Likewise, most tests were only performed in a qualitative manner. However, as more procedures were developed using 'wet ashing' and the Stas–Otto technique some quantitative procedures also began to appear. Quantita-tive methods for alcohol were introduced in 1852 by Cotte based on the reduction of chromic acid. Electrolytic deposition techniques for metals were first used in 1862. In 1879, a method for the quantitation of arsenic was devised by Gutzeit. A quantitative procedure for carbon monoxide using palladium chloride reduction was introduced in 1880 by Fodor. Quantitative methods for alkaloids were introduced in 1890.

In 1918, New York replaced its coroners' system with the Medical Examiner's Office after members of the New York Academy of Medicine demonstrated that the medicolegal investigations carried out by politically-appointed coroners were not adequate to protect the public's interest. A toxicology laboratory was established immediately. The chief forensic toxicologist of this laboratory was Alexander O. Gettler, the 'Father of American Toxicology'. During the first 30 years of the laboratory, the only analytical instruments were a Doboscq colorimeter, and analytical balance, a pH meter, a filter photometer, and a van Slyke manometric gas analysis apparatus. Despite the lack of the existence of more sophisticated analytical equipment, the laboratory was able to analyse biolgicals for alcohol, cyanide, fluoride, carbon monoxide poisonings, thallium, and the micro-isolation of volatile toxic substances from tissue.

Professional Organizations, Certification and Instrumentation

In 1949 the American Academy of Forensic Sciences was formed to promote the practice of the forensic sciences, including foresic toxicology. Since that time several other organizations have been formed which have only forensic toxicologists as members. Two such organizations are the International Association of Forensic Toxicologists (1963) and the Society of Forensic Toxicologists (1970).

The three decades from 1960 to 1990 has seen an astronomical growth in technology applied to the science of forensic toxicology. Sophisticated instrumentation incuding thin-layer chromatography, spectophotometry, gas chromatography, immunoassays, mass spectrometry and high-pressure liquid chromatography have all been applied successfully to analyses in the area of forensic toxicology. These analytical techniques will be discussed below.

Until the early 1980s forensic toxicology was primarily concerned with medical examiners' cases and blood alcohol concentrations (BACs) in driving under the influence (DUI) cases. However, with the advent of testing for drugs in the armed services and the workplace, the birth of a new area of forensic toxiclology occurred, Forensic Urine Drug Testing (FUDT). The demand for 'certified' forensic toxicologists to direct 'certified forensic urine drug testing laboratories' has caused a shortage of 'Board Certified Forensic Toxicologists' in the US. Toxicology certification is available from several sources including the American Board of Forensic Toxicology and the American Association of Clinical Chemists. In other countries similar qualifications are available, e.g., the Diploma in Forensic Pathology of the Royal College of Pathologists in the UK. Another new frontier in the 1980s for forensic toxicologists has been the testing for driving under the influence of drugs other than alcohol (DUID). This chapter will focus on traditional post-mortem forensic toxicology.

The Forensic Laboratory

The forensic toxicology laboratory is responsible for demonstrating the absence or presence of chemical substances in biological and non-biological specimens in connection with medicolegal investigations. The laboratory must be capable of analysing a wise variety of toxic substances. Alcohol, antidepressants, barbiturates, bezodiazepines (minor tranquillizers), carbon monoxide, chlorinated hydrocarbons, cocaine, heavy metals (arsenic, antimony, bismuth and mercury), insecticides, lead, opium alkaloids, non-barbiturate sedative hypnotics, phenothazines, and stimulants are among the most frequently encountered substances in the forensic laboratory.

The toxicology laboratory is responsible for the handling of evidence and must maintain a proper chain of evidence with receipts or records for the transfer and storage of materials to be analysed. The specimens should be properly refrigerated until transported to the laboratory. Specimens must be delivered to the laboratory with proper identification of the specimen affixed to each container. The information on the container label should include the name of the deceased, the case number, date of sampling and the type of sample. When the specimens are delivered to the laboratory, they must be accompanied by a proper transmittal form that shows the name, case number, date and types of specimens being transmitted. Any discrepancies in the form and the samples should be noted on the transmittal form and signed and dated by the receiving person in the laboratory and the person making the delivery. Additional documentation includes: a laboratory work sheet and a report form.

Specimen Storage

Ideally, storage capacity should be adequate to store all specimens indefinitely. This idea is impractical because storage space is usually limited. A written policy must be established concerning disposal of samples. The policy should include the effective date of the policy, the length of time specimens will be held and a mechanism by which a request can be made for an extension of storage. A reasonable length of storage is 2 years; this will allow for adjudication of most court proceedings, both criminal and civil.

Specimens are usually kept refrigerated (4°C) during the time they are being analysed (short-term storage) and then in a freezer (–10°C) until disposed of (long-term storage). It has been calculated that approximately 0.85 cubic metres of freezer space is required to store the specimens from 500 cases.

The Forensic Toxicologist

The role of the forensic toxicologist in the forensic investigations is to determine whether various toxicants were present or absent in the specimens submitted to the laboratory. He must be a firstrate analytical chemist and be knowledgeable about the effects of poisons. He must know the 'older' techniques in addition to the newly evolving ones.

The major responsibilities of the forensic toxicologist include: on the-scene investigation, preservation of chains of evidence (external and internal), oral and written reports, consultation (pathologist, police, attorneys), expert testimony, research and development, education (self and others) and above all the ability to interpret the meaning of the concentration of the toxicant. The absence of a particular toxicant may be as important to a particular case as the detection of the substance in lethal concentrations. For example, finding subtherapeutic concentrations of antipathetic drugs is important in convulsion-related deaths. The presence of low concentrations of carboxyhaemoglobin in a suspected fire death always raises questions about the actual cause of death.

The forensic toxicologist is responsible for all the results that are reported by the laboratory. He must be familiar with all the procedures used by the laboratory and capable of developing new methods when they are needed. He must recognize that all laboratories have analytical limitations and be knowledgeable of when and where outside sources should be utilized.

The forensic toxicologists must have the proper educational background and professional experience necessary to interpret the laboratory's results. He must be knowledgable of the specificity and sensitivity of the equipment and procedures utilized in the analyses. The forensic toxicologist must be capable of defending the results in judicial proceedings to a reasonable degree of medical and scientific certainty. His reputation will be reinforced by his work record, evidence of professional growth through peer reviewed publications, presentations at professional meetings, membership of professional societies, and 'Board Certifications' in the USA, and equivalent in other countries.

One must always remember that the most important criteria in the interpretation of results are the circumstances surrounding the death. In the case of a low carboxy-haemoglobin in the above mentioned example, it would be important to know if the fire victim had been given oxygen or had been doused with petrol (gasoline). In either of these circumstances the carboxyhaemoglobin might be less than 10 per cent of total haemoglobin. Another example in which the toxicology results help to complete the circumstances is as follows: a person was last seen alive 6 hours prior to his body being found with a gunshot wound to the back of his head. When last seen he was sharing a marijuana joint with his friend. Analysis of the blood of the deceased revealed a concentration of 60 ng ml^{-1} of delat-9-THC and 100 ng ml^{-1} of THC-Acid. This result would indicate that the person had died less than 1–2 hours after smoking the marijuana cigarette. This type of information aids in the investigation and helps to narrow the time of death estimation.

Even in cases where circumstances make the cause of death obvious the laboratory may be able to solve some questions such as was the homicide drug-related; was the deceased sexually molested (acid phosphatase); did the person jump out the window because he was 'high' on some type of drug (PCP, LSD, etc.).

Specimens

As the autopsy usually occurs before the investigation into circumstances surrounding the case is final, it is important to obtain adequate types and volumes of specimens at the time of the autopsy. The specimens collected in a specific medical examiner's case may differ depending on the circumstances. However, in all medicolegal investigation cases a blood specimen should be obtained when blood is available. The analysis of a post-mortem specimen is only as reliable as the conditions surrounding its collection (Plueckhahn, 1968). Proper collection of specimens often requires the addition of preservatives and/ or enzyme poisons to protet the specimen from post-mortem changes, such as bacterial production of ethanol or other alcohols or their loss. A commonly employed agent for this purpose is sodium fluoride at a concentration of at least 10 mg ml^{-1} of specimen.

Traditionally heart blood has been collected at autopsy. However, recent studies have shown with drugs like propoxyphene, tricyclic anti-depressants (amitriptyline, imipramine, doxepin, etc.) and many others that heart blood concentrations can increase post-mortem (Andrenyak and Backer, 1988; Bandt, 1981; Jones, 1986; Proutry and Anderson, 1984, 1990). Some reports show a relationship between post-mortem interval (time from death to autopsy) and concentration increase (Bandt, 1981; Jones, 1986; Prouty and Anderson, 1984, 1990). This concentration difference in heart blood and other peripheral sites is referred to as 'anatomical site concentration differences' or 'post-mortem redistribution'. Peripheral blood concentrations have been shown to be more reliable with these drugs when compared with peri-mortem concentrations (Andrenyak and Backer, 1988; Apple and Bandt, 1988; Prouty and Anderson, 1984, 1990). Therefore, in all suspected drug overdoses or in cases of unknown causes of death a femoral blood specimen should be collected and analysed.

It is also interest that some drugs even within the same specimen do not show an increase while others do. The carisoprodol heart/femoral concentration ratio (H/F) was 1.02 and the propoxyphene H/F was 2.03. Other authors have proposed that drug concentrations in liver specimens are a better indicator of toxicity (Apple and Bandt, 1988; Prouty and Anderson, 1990; Roetlger, 1990).

Some studies have reported that heart blood alcohol concentrations also change during the post-mortem interval (Bowden and McCallum, 1949; Turkle and Gifford, 1957; Briglia *et al.*, 1986). The authors of these studies recommend that femoral blood specimens be used for alcohol determinations in post-mortem cases. In several other studies it has been shown that heart blood concentrations of alcohol did not change post mortem in intact bodies and that concentration differences of ethanol in heart and femoral blood are minor and more likely represent the expected differences seen in the absorptive phases of alcohol consumption (Plueckhahn, 1968; Backer *et al.*, 1980; Prouty and Anderson, 1984). However, in case where bacterial infiltration of the body is likely a femoral specimen is recommended.

Procedural Approach

The particular approach that a laboratory takes for testing biological specimens is dictated by the type of services it provides. Therefore, a laboratory serving a hospital emergency room will be interested in rapid turnaround time for the common drugs of abuse. Laboratories testing for chemical substances to determine the cause of death typically utilize a large variety of different types of tests including screening tests, chromatographic methods (spectrophot-metric, thin-layer gas, mass spectrometry, high-pressure liquid chromatography) and immunoassays. The postmortem forensic laboratory must be prepared to analyse for a number of commonly encountered analytes.

Types of Testing

Colorimetric Screening Test

Screening tests are usually performed directly on biological specimens with little or no sample preparation (Widdop, 1986). Some of the most common substances tested for include phenothiazines, imipramine, desipramine, trimipramine, halogenated compounds, salicaylates, paracetamol (acetaminophen), ethchlorvynol and heavy metals (Gettler and Kaye, 1950). These tests are rapid and informative but only presumptive. As many of them only identify a class of compounds, they usually require further identification of the specific toxicant and confirmation.

Steam Distillation

Volatile substances can be separated from blood, urine or tissue homogenates by steam distillation. The specimen is made either acidic with hydrochloric acid or basic with solid magnesium oxide. Steam is poassed into the solution and the aqueous distillate collected by condensation. Analytes dislikable from acidic solutions include ethanol, methanol, phenols, halogenated hydrocarbons, cyanide and ethchlorvynol. Distilliates from basic solutions will contain volatile basic drugs such as amphetamines, meperidine, methadone and nicotine. The distillates can then be analysed by various techniques including colorimetric tests, immunoassays, spectroscopy and various chromatographic methods including thin-layer, gas and liquid chromatography.

Micordiffusion

Microdiffusion is a convenient, rapid separation technique that allows for the analyte to be either detected as it is isolated (alcohols, carbon monoxide) or to be captured in an appropriate medium and tested by various techniques (cyanide, meethoal, phenols, chlorinated hydrocarbons, sulphides). The technique of isolation utilizes a Conway microdiffusion dis. A comprehensive review of microdicusion applications has been described in the literature. A microdiffusion method for ethchlorvynol has also been described (Peel and Freimuth, 1972).

Spectroscocpy

Spectorscopy is based on the principle that substances either gain or lose energy when subjected to electromagnetic radiation. Identification of the substance may be possible by noting the wavelengths at which the energy change takes place. The energy changes are proportional to the quantity of the analyte present and therefore the method can also be used for qunatitation. The common types of spectroscopy utilized in the forensic laboratory include visible, ultraviolet, fluormetry, atomic absorption and infrared.

Chromatography

Chromatography is a separation technique utilizing a partitioning process. Mixtures of drugs and their metabolites are commonly separated by chromatography. Chromatogrphy requires a stationary or fixed phase, which may be a liquid or solid absorbed on an inert support having a large surface area, and a moving or mobile phase of a liquid or gas. In a chromatographic method, analytes within a mixture are moved by the mobile phase while the different interactions of the individual analytes with the stationary phase cause separation from other components. After separation the components are identified by various means including colorimetric, electrolytic, and/or spectrophotometric.

Most chromotographic techniques require an extraction of the specimen before analysis. The extent of the 'clean-up' prior to chromatography depends on many variables including the nature of the matrix, the concentration of the analyte of interests and the type of chromatography. Liquid-liquid extraction is one of the most common separation techniques. Other types of extraction techniques commonly employed include liquid-solid such as charcoal, and solid phase extractions.

Thin-Layer Chromatography (TLC)

This is a rather simple separation technique which does not require a lot of expensive equipment. An extract of a biological specimen is applied as a concentrated spot at the origin of a TLC plate. The plate is placed in a developing tank with just enough solvent to submerge the bottom 1–1.5 cm. As the solvent (mobile phase) moves up the plate by capillary action, drugs and their metabolites are separated depending on the polarity of the solvent system and the solubility characteristics of the compounds in the extract. Visualization is accomplished with colour reagents and long- and short-wave ultraviolet light. The distance the compound travelled from the origin divided by the distance the solvent travelled from the origin is called the R_f or migration value. The R_f value along with the colour reactions are used for qualitative and semi-qunatitative results.

In general, TLC is a fairly sensitive technique. The specificity of TLC can be increased by using multiple chromatogenic sprays. Most spray reagents are non-destructive and the analytes can be removed and tested by other anlytical techniques. The major disadvantages of TLC include the need for extraction prior to analysis and that the experience of the chromatographer will affect the quality of the results. Some excellent reviews of different TLC separation and visualization techniques can be found in the literature.

With some drugs a confirmation test can be performed directly on the TLC plate or the spot after removal without further extraction. A procedure for pethidine confirmation by fluorometry directly on TLC spots without extraction is described below. The spot corresponding to pethidine is removed with a spatula and placed in a 10 ml beaker and then processed as follows. To the TLC scarpings add 5 drops of Marquis reagent (8–10 drops of 40 per cent formaldehyde in 10 ml concentrated sulphuric acid) and heat in an oven at 110°C for 10 min. Then add 1 ml distilled water and observe under long-wave ultraviolet light. A blue fluorescence indicates that pethidine may be present. To confirm its presence, and 2 ml of water and scan in a spectrofluorometer, excitation 270 μm, emission 420 and 440 μm.

TLC drug identification systems can be purchased from commercial sources. One system, Toxi-LAB, available from Analytical Systems, Irvine, California, utilizes silica-gel impreganted paper and dips rather than sprays for visualization. Its chromatogram is subjected to four visualization steps (stages), the colours and R_f values are noted for each stage for hundreds of drugs are supplied by the manufacturer. The advantage of this type of system is that it makes everything available including extraction tubes, visualization reagents, the photocompendium, confirmation systems, drug standards, continula updates on new drugs, and technical assitance. The disadvantage is the cost, but much of that is offset by technician time savings in not having to prepare visualization reagents, extraction tubes, and less technical training necessary to be proficient at identification. The identification process is also available on computer disk.

Gas Liquid Chromatography (GLC)

Like TLC, GLC is a separation technique. It is one of the most widely used techniques for drug analysis, for both screening and confirmation procedures. It uses an inert gas, such as nitrogen or helium as the mobile phase. An extract of the biological specimen is dissolved in a small amount of organic solvent (usually 25–100 μl) and then injected into a heated injector. The sample is vaporized and swept on to the column by the carrier gas (mobile phase). The identification of compounds in GLC is by retention time.

The column is in an oven with a temperature controller. The vaporized sample is carried through the column by a controlled flow rate of the mobile phase. The stationary phase interacts with the sample causing the analytes within the mixture to separate. The retention time is a measure of the elapsed time from the injection of the extract into the gas chromatograph until the apex of the detector response.

A column's capability to separate analytes can be modified by using different types and amounts of liquid phases (stationary phases) absorbed on an inert solid phase. Types of columns used include packed and capillary columns. Packed columns are usually glass, 1–2 metres in length and 3–6 mm in diameter. Capillary columns usually offer better separation than packed columns. They are commonly made of fused silica, 10–100 metres in length and have a diameter of between 0.25 and 0.60 mm. The stationary phase is a thin film (usually 0.25–1.0 µm).

Gas Chromatography/Mass Spectrometry (GC/MS)

GC/MS combines the separating powers of the gas chromatograph with the discriminating abilities of a mass spectrometer. This combination of instrumentation (GC/MS) is recognized as the most defnitive method of identification of a drug in a biological specimen and is the current benchmark of positive identification.

The basic operation of a mss spectrometer can be separated into three steps:

(1) ionization,

(2) mass filtration and

(3) detection.

The most common mode of operation mass spectrometer utilizes electron impact (EI) for ionization. Neutral molecules in a gas phase are bombarded with high energy electrons which causes the molecules to lose an electron, therefore carrying a positive charge and sufficient energy to undergo fragmentation. The fragmentation pattern always occurs in the same manner thereby creating an identifiable spectrum. The spectrum fragmentation pattern for a given compound is its fingerprint.

Another mode of mass spectrometer operation is selective ion monitoring (SIM). In this mode the MS monitors the ion current of only those ions of a few masses that are characteristic for a for a specific drug. SIM affords a higher sensitivity for most mass spectrometers, but provides a less specific pattern for identification. Other modes of operation include 'positive and negative' chemical ionization (CI). The spectra produced from CI are typically less complex and more sensitive than EI spectra.

Liquid Chromatography (LC)

LC is one of the oldest anlytical separation techniques. The technique was a slow separation process when first developed because the mobile phase flowed through a column by gravity only. Modern techniques referred to as high-performance liquid chromatography (HPLC) utilize pumps to pass the mobile phases through columns at pressures exceeding 1000 psi. The major components of a basic high-performance liquid chromatograph are a solvent reservior (mobile phase), a pump, a packed column (the stationary phase) and a detector. There are several different types of detectors including spectrophotometric, electrochemical, fluorescence and mass spectrometric. The characteristic measurement used in HPLC is time from injection to detection at a given flow rate. Additional specificity can be added by the type of detectors, on-line ultraviolet analysis, or by using different wavelengths for detection.

This technique has become widespread in clinical toxicology and is becoming more popular in foresnsic work. Recent reports have been published on the use of HPLC in forensic cases involving benzodiazepines and marijuana.

Immunoassays

Immunoassays are based on a competition between the drug of interest in the specimen and a 'labelled, drug added to the specimen for sites on an antibody for the drug of interest.

Enzyme Immunoassay (EIA)

EIA is a homogeneous enzyme technique, the antigen (drug) and antibody complex does not need to be separated from the matrix before assaying. The EIA system most often described is the EMIT system (Syva Corporation, Palo Alto, California). In the EMIT assay, the label on the antigen (drug) is an enyzme. The specimen to be tested, usually urine, is mixed with a reagent containing glucose 6-phosphate (G-6-P) and antibodies to the drug of interest. A second reagent containing a derivative of the drug labelled with G-6-P dehydrogenase is added to the specimen. The enzyme is inactive when bound to an antibody site. If the drug in interest or its metabolite were present in the specimen then it will also react with the limited number of antibodies. This would have the effect of increasing the activity of the enzyme and allows for a semi-quantitative measurement of the concentration of the drug and/or it is metabolite. A recent study has shown by using a 5-point calibration curve and a logit data transform that reasonable quantitation of some drugs with EIA is possible (Standefer *et al.,* 1989).

The advantages of EIA include a short analysis time and minimal sample preparation. The sensitivity is adequate for most drugs of abuse. Disadvantages of the system include the tests not being specific and the cost of reagents.

Radiommunoassays (RIA)

RIA is also a competitive reaction for antibody sites between a drug and/or its metbolites and a radioactive labelled drug. After separation of the antigen–antibody complex the radioactivity is determined on either the supernatant or the precipitated antibody. The presence or absence of the drug is indicated by the radioactivity of the sample. If the supernatant is counted, a positive specimen is one in which the radioactivity counts are equal to or greater than a standard. When the precipitate is counted, a positive specimen is indicated when the radioactive counts are equal to or less than those of a standard. The advantages of RIA are its sensitivity and small sample size. The disadvantages are incubation time, need for radioactive materials, and cost of reagents.

Fluorescent Polarization Immunoassays (FPI)

FPI utilizes a drug labelled with a fluorescent substance. The labelled drug competes with the unlabelled drug or metabolite in the specimen for an anitbody site. When a fluorophore is excited by polarized light it will emit polarized light. A larger molecule will emit a greater proportion of polarized light. The antibody–fluorescent-labelled drug complex results in a macromolecule and therefore an increased fluorescence. The amount of drug and/or metabolite in the specimen is inversely related to the amount of fluorescent polarization. The advantage of the technique is its sensitivity. The major disadvantage is the cost of the reagents.

Analytical Schemes for The Detection of Poisons

The major types of medicolegal cases include apparent natural causes of death, accidents (motor vehicle related), accidents (non-motor vehicle related), homicides, suicides, and drug abuse. The circumstances surrounding the case will usually determine the types of toxicology tests that are required. In almost all cases a volatile screen (VS) will be required. Other types of protocols include a Drugs of Abuse Screen (DAS), a General Drug Screen (GDS), an Acidic/Neutral Screen (ANS), and a Basic Drug Screen (BDS).

The most frequently requested test in a forensic toxicology laboratory is a volatile screen (VS) for ethanol. There are many different types of techniques available for ethanol analysis such as oxidiative, enzymatic or gas chromatographic. The most popular method in forensic applications for determining ethanol is GLC. GLC has the ability to separate commonly encountered volatiles including ethanol, methanol, acetone, and isopropanol providing the required specificity and sensitivity to measure ethanol as low as 2.2 mmol l^{-1} (10 mg dl^{-1}). A typical GLC procedure, using flame ionization detection (FID) for ethanol would employ an internal standard such as *n*-propanol or *t*-butyl alcohol. The peak height or areas reasponses of etahnol to the internal standard would be compared with a series of aqueous standards with the same amount of internal standard for quantitation. Direct injection analysis procedures for alcohols have been described (Jain, 1971; Winek and Carfagna, 1987) as well as head space procedures using both packed columns (Dubowski, 1977) and capillary columns (Penton, 1987).

There are instances when a suitable blood specimen is not available for anlaysis (such as traumatic injuries) or when the body is decomposing. Endogenous (post-mortem neoformation) production of alcohol is a well-known occurrence (Blackmore, 1968). In cases where a suitable blood specimen is not available it may be possible to analyse various other biological specimens and at least make an estimate of the blood concentration (Backer *et al.,* 1980). Vitreous humor has been shown to be a fluid useful in the determination of alcohol in the absence of blood and in decomposing bodies (Coe, 1972; Zumwalt *et al.,* 1982). The finding of ethanol in the vitreous humor and/or urine of a cadaver is consistent with an exogenous (ingested before death) source of alcohol. In Zumwalt's study of 130 decomposing bodies the highest concentration of endogenous ethanol was 47.8 mmol l^{-1} (220 mg dl^{-1}).

Another problem in ethanol determinations arises in embalmed cases. Embalming fluid can contain ethanol (Winek, 1984) and the embalming process has been reported to reduce the ethanol concentration by 52 per cent when it is free of ethanol (Bronstein and Park, 1984; Backer, 1989). Ethanol concentratons in vitreous humor have been shown to be useful in embalmed cases. In a series of cases where pre-embalmed and post-embalmed vitreous alcohol concentrations were determined (Coe, 1976; Scott *et al.,* 1974), 78 per cent of the time the post-embalmed concentration was within 6.5 mmol l^{-1} (30 mg dl^{-1}) of the usually higher pre-embalmed specimen's ethanol concentration.

A Drugs of Abuse Screen (DAS) commonly tests for amphetamines, barbiturates, benzodiazepines, cocaine, marijuana, methadone, propoxyphene, phencyclidine and opiate alkaloids. The DAS should be requested in most homicides and accidental deaths. The most common methodology for a DAS is an enzyme immunoassay (EIA) usually performed on urine but applicable to other specimens.

A General Drug Screen (GDS) is a broad spectrum analysis for many drugs and is necessary when the cause of death is not clear. The GDS is usually a TLC method and is applicable to many different specimens including urine, blood, gastric and tissue homogenates.

The Acidic and Neutral Drug Screen (ANS) is usually a GC (GC/MS) method for acidic drugs and neutral drugs including barbiturates and nonbarbiturate sedative hyponotics such as glutethimide and muscle relaxants including meprobamate and carisoprodol. The ANS method is applicable to many types of specimens including blood, urine and tissue homogenates.

The Basic Drug Screen (BDS) is usually a GC (GC/MS) method for the analysis of many basic drugs such as propoxyphene, cocaine, antidepressants, opiates (codeine, oxycodone, hydromorphone, meperidine), calcium channel blockers, and many others.

Miscellaneous protocols that are also needed for other commonly encountered analytes include cyanide, carboxyhaemo-globin, arsenic and other metals, pesticides, aromatic, aliphatic and chlorinated hydrocarbons, and vitreous chemistries such as sodium, chloride and glucose. There are many different published texts that can be referred to for protocols to analyse these and other anlaytes (Sunshine, 1971; Moffat *et al.,* 1986; Baselt and Cravey, 1989).

Interpretation of Results

After the analyses of specimens for a particular case are complete, the forensic toxicologist must interpret the findings as to the physilogical effects of the analytes in retrospect to their concentrations. The specific questions that must be answered are whether the concentrations of any analyte or combinations of analytes were:

* sufficient to cause the death?
* sufficient to have affected the actions of the decedent so as to have caused the death?
* insufficient to have any involvement in the cause of death?
* insufficient to protect the individual from an underlying mechanism of death such as an epileptic seizure?

Many factors must be taken into account including the route of administration. The most common methods of administration of toxicants are oral, intravenous and inhalation. As the concentrations of drugs administered intravenously that result in fatalities are quite often much less than found in oral overdoses it can be very important to know the route. In forensic cases the route may not always be known unless evidence is found at the scene such as a syringe and the decedent has very recent injection sites. The toxicology finding may answer some questions about the route, for example, finding a large amount of drug or even intact medication in the stomach contents is a good indication of an oral route of administration. However, some drugs are absorbed very rapidly, such as tricyclic antidepressants, and even when massive overdoses are ingested only traces may be found in the gastric contents. It is important to point out that with most analytes the presence of the drug in the gastric contents is not sufficient proof that it was the agent or one of a combination of toxicants that caused the death. It must be documented that suffcient absorption of the substance occured to result in a toxic concentration of the analyte in blood and/or liver. Other findings such as extremely high lung concentrations of a drug or chemical are very suggestive of an inhalation route.

It has always been assumed that the concentration of most analytes in heart blood paralleled the physiological consequences. This premise had been shown to be untrue in recent years (Prouty and Anderson, 1989, 1990; Jones and Pounder, 1987; Andrenyak and Bakcer, 1988). It is now known that the concentration of many analytes increases in both heart and peripheral blood specimens during the post-mortem interval. These anatomical site concentration differences have shown that in most cases femoral blood is more liekly to be a better indicator of the perimortem (at death) concentration of the analyte. Reference to common tabulations of toxic concentrations of analytes (Winek, 1976; Baselt *et al.*, 1975; Baselt and Cravey, 1977; Stead and Moffat, 1983) must be used with extreme caution because most are based on heart blood findings. The liver concentration and/or brain concentration of an analyte may be extremely important in the determination of the involvement of an analyte in the cause of death. The toxic concentrations of many analytes in liver can be found in tabular form (McBay, 1973; Baselt and Cravey, 1977). The concentration ratios of the analyte in blood to liver are often very helpful in interpretation of the involvement of the analyte (Stajic *et al.*, 1979). With some drugs like methadone the therapeutic (or maintenance concentration) overlaps the concentrations found in overdoses. However, it has been postulated that the concentration ratio of 1,5-dimethyl-3,3-diphenyl-2-ethylidenepyrrolidine, a major metabolite of methadone, in liver to kidney is always less than or equal to 1 in an overdose of methadone (Thompson, 1976). The ratio of blood propoxyphene, has also been investigated in predicting toxicity.

Drugs taken in combination can be more toxic than if considered separately. Knowledge of the interaction of toxicants will be paramount to proper interpretation of the toxicity of any analyte. Most analytes are more toxic in the the presence of alcohol. The toxicity of barbiturates and alcohol has been studied (Cimbura *et al.*, 1972). Unfortunately, information about most combinations of analytes is not well known and the toxicologist must quite often deal with them on an individual basis. Experience with similar cases or published reports will be the only information the forensic toxicologist can rely on in predicting the toxicity of many analyte combinations.

Other factors that must be considered in the

interpretative process by the forensic toxicologist are the age, sex, body weight, genetic factors, tolerance, environmental exposures and general health status of the individual. All of these factors can influence the response to a given concentration of an analyte or combinations of analytes. Liver disease may prevent the metabolism of an analyte allowing multiple dosing to result in accumulation of the drug to toxic concentrations, or an underlying condition such as atherosclerotic cardiovascular disease will make the presence of an analyte at a given concentration more toxic. Environmental exposure as well as abusive uses of halogenated hydrocarbons can result in sensitization or myocardial tissues, making an individual more susceptible to a cardiac arrhythmia (Reinhardt *et al.*, 1971).

Conclusion

Post-mortem forensic toxicology has changed dramatically in the past 20 years. Some of the major changes have been related to analytical techniques such as immunoassays, high-performance liquid chromatography and the role of gas chromatography/mass spectrometry in positive identification of toxicants. The knowledge that the concentrations of many drugs are not stable post morten has also caused considerbale debate and change in the toxicologist's ability to interpret his analytical findings.

2

Epidemiology in Relation to Toxicology

Introduction

Epidemiology is sometimes simply defined as the study of patterns of health in groups of people (Paddle, 1988). Behind this deceptively simple definition lies a surprisingly diverse science, rich in concepts and methodology. For instance, the group of people might consist of only two people. Goudie *et al.*, (1985) described a father suffering from rheumatiod arthritis and his daughter with vertigo. In both father and daughter the pattern of affected areas was remarkably similar, which might suggest that the distribution of joint lesions in rheumatiod arthritis is genetically determined. At the opposite extreme, studies of the geomgraphic distribution of diseases using national mortality and cancer incidence rates have provided clues about the aetiology of several diseases such as cardiovascular disease and stomach cancer. The patterns of health studied are also wide-ranging, and may include the distribution, course and spread of disease. The term 'disease' also has a loose definition in the context of epidemiology, and might include ill-defined conditions such as Organic Solvent and Sick Building Syndromes or consist of an indirect measure of impairment such as biochemical and haematological parameters or lung function measurements.

McMadhon and Pugh (1970) observe that epidemiology has evolved from the study of striking outbreaks of disease or epidemićs, and note that modern epidemiology can still be regarded as the study of epidmics if a broad view is taken as to what constitutes an epidemic. Clearly epdiemiology has a very wide scope, but the aim of this chapter is to describe the relationship between epidemiology and toxicology. For this reason, discussion will be mainly limited to the role epidemiology plays alongside toxicology in the assessment of the hazards of chemical and physical agents and the recommendation of safe conditions under which we may come into contact with them.

Both toxicology and epidemiology are considered by many to be relatively new scientific disciplines. Toxicology, however, has a longer tradition and in the twentieth century it has come to be regarded as a science in its own right and not simply a branch of pharmacology. In order to survivie, our prehistoric ancestors had to be aware which foods were harmful, and they were naturally led to exeriment in order to cure natural ailments or develop antidotes to poisons. There is evidence that poisons were used for hunting and fishing and that prehistoric man was aware of the therapeutic benefits of certain natural substances. There are many early examples of toxicological writings such as the Papyrus Ebers of the ancient Egyptians, written about 1500 BC, and the Sanskrit medical writings in the Ayur Veda, which date back to around 900 BC. Decker (1987) provides a good description of the early history of the science of poisons and the rapid development of analytical toxicology during the nineteenth and twentieth centuries. In contrast, epidemiologists can quote Hippocrates to demostrate that the ancient Greeks were aware that health may be connected with a person's environment.

However, there the similarity with toxicology ends, for it was not until the seventeenth century that the beginnings of quantitative epidemiology started to appear. John Graunt, who in 1662 published his *Natural and Political*

Observations...on the Bills of Mortality, is often credited as being the pioneer of quantitative epidemiology, although McMahon and Pugh (1970) note that, since the techniques of Graunt saw no further epidemiological application for almost 200 years, it is more appropriate to regard Graunt as a forerunner than a founder of epidemiology. Although the nineteenth century saw important work by people such as William Farr and John Snow, most of the theory and quantitative methods of epidemiology have really only come into being during the past four decades.

Epidemiology and toxicology differ in many other ways but principally in that epidemiology is essentially an observational science, in contrast to the experimental nature of toxicology. The opportunistic approach of epidemiology has been commented upon by several authors (e.g., Paddle, 1988; Utidjian, 1987). The epidemiologist often has to make to with historical data which have been collected for reasons which have nothing to do with epidemiology. Nevertheless, the availability of personnel records such as lists of new starters and leavers, payrolls and work rosters and exposure monitoring data collected for compliance purposes has enabled many epidemiological studies to be conducted in the occupational setting. Thus, the epidemiologist has no control over who is exposed to an agent, the levels at which they are exposed to the agent of interest, or other agents to which they may be exposed. The epidemilogist has great difficulty in ascertaining what exposure has taken place and certainly has no control over life-style variables such as diet and smoking.

Despite the lack of precise data, the epidemiologist has one major advatage over the toxicologist: an epidemiology study documents the actual health experiences of human beings subjected to real-life exposures in an occupational or environmental setting. Indeed Smith (1988) has recently expressed the view that uncertainty in epidemiology studies resulting from exposure estimation may be equal to or less than the uncertainty associated with extrapolation from animals to man. Regulatory bodies such as the US

Environmental Protection Agency (EPA) are starting to change their attitudes towards epidemiology and recognize that it has a role to play in the process of risk assessment. However, there is also a complementary need for epidemiologists to introduce more rigour into the conduct of their studies and to introduce standards akin to the Good Laboratory Practice standards under which animal experiments are performed.

History of Epidemiology

As noted in the introduction, awareness of certain epidemiological principles can be traced back to the days of Hippocrates, but it was a further 2000 years before epidemiology truly began to emerge. The anlysis by John Graunt of the weekly Bills of Mortality and christenings recorded in the parish registers of London is generally regarded to be the first example of an epidemiological study. He reported higher death rates and birth rates for males than for females, and examined the influence of various factors on the spread of plague. However, the greatest achievement of Graunt was to recognize the importance of studying biological phenomena in groups people. Edmund Halley, the English Astronomer Royal, was another seventeenth century scientist who was intrested in population mortality rates. Healley made a study of the records of births and deaths kept in the Silesian city of Breslau (now Wroclaw in Poland) since 1584 and drew up a life-table which was published in 1693. Casina Stable, a seventeenth century Italian physician, has received comparatively little recognition. However, the following extract from *De Morbis Artificum* (*Diseas of Workers*) written by Ramazzini in 1713 (Ramazzini, 1964), demonstrates clearly that Stabe understood the basic principles of epidemiology:

A few years ago a violent dispute arose between a citizen of Finale, a town in the dominion of Modena, and a certain business man, a Modenese, who owned a huge laboratory at Finale where he manufactured sublimate. The sitizen of Finale brought a lawsuit against this manufacturer and demanded that he should move his workship outside the town or to some other place, on the ground that he poisoned the whole neighbourhodd whenever his workmen roasted vitroil in the furnace to make sublimate. To prove the truth of his accusation he produced the sworn testimony of the doctor of Finale and also the parish registrer of deaths, from which it appeared that many more persons died annually in that quarter and in the immediate neigbourhood of the laboratory than in other localities. Moreover, the doctor gave evidence that the residents of that neighbourhood usually died of wasting disease and disease of the chest; this he ascribed to the fumes given off by the vitriol, which so tainted the air near by that it was rendered unhealthy and dangerous for the lungs. Dr. Bernardino Corradi, the commissioner of ordnance in the Duchy of Este, defended the manufacture, while Dr Casina Stable, then the twon physician, spoke for the plaintiff. Various cleverly worded documents were published by both sides, and this dispute which was literally 'about the shadow of smoke', as the saying is, was hotly argues. In the end the jury sustained the manufacturer, and vitriol was found not guilty. Whether in this case the legal expert gave a correct verdict, I leave to the decision of those who are experts in natural science.

During the nineteenth century modern epidemiological theory began to take shape. In 1836 the registration of births, marriages and deaths became compusory in England, and William Farr, appointed Registrar General for England and Wales in 1839, established a pattern for the reporting of mortality data which has continued to this day. Farr looked at mortality in a variety of occupational settings and established a procedure for linking mortality data to occupational groupings derived from census data. A Parisain physican who taught Farr, Pierre-Charles Alexandre Louis, is given much credit for introducing numerical techniques to occupational epidemiology (Lilienfeld and Lilienfeld, 1977). louis also taught another eminent Victorain epdiemiologist, William Guy (see Weed, 1986, for a discussion of some of Guy's work). Another Victorain pioneer in epidemiology was John Snow, who was famous for demostrating the relationship between the incidence of cholera in certain London boroughs and faecal contamination of the water supply. McMahon and Pugh (1970) give a more detailed description of the work of Farr and Snow. The work of Farr and Snow is extremely well known but there were also many other excellent epidemiological studies conducted during the nineteenth century. Florence Nightingale, well known as the Lady of the Lamp, was also a reformer who knew how medical statistics could benefit her causes. She was a firm friend of William Farr, and one example of her work was a mortality table for hospital nurses and attendants showing a greatly increased prevalence of communicable diseases (Newell, 1984).

This progress continued into the twentieth centruy, and Utidjian (1987) points out that during the early years of the twentieth century there were a number of important occupational morbidity studies. In addition, there was much work done by acturaries in the insurance business which is often overlooked and predates the conventional landmarks of classical epidemiology. After the pioneering work of Graunt and Halley it was a further generation before James Dodson laid the foundations of actuarial science. Dodson calculated a scale of premiums based on the Bills of Mortality for London in the years 1728–1750. The life insurance business then developed steadily over the next 150 years. From the beginning of the twentieth century, the insurance companies of the USA and Canada have conducted many large-seale investigations of the mortality associated with various impariments. The first large scale mortality study by the insurance companies, reported in 1903, *The Specialised Mortality Investigation,* was notable in that the results were reported as mortailitg ratios.

Having given due recognition to the nineteenth century fathers of epidemiology such as Farr and Snow, it is still fair to say that epidemiology has only begun to develop as a science in the last 40 years. Greenland (1987), writing about the evolution of epidemiological ideas, stated that the period from World War II up to the early 1980s encompasses the two 'golden eras' of epidemiological development. In Greenland's view, a foundation for epidemiological research was created during the years 1946–1966 and this coincided with the conduct of the first major studies of chronic disease. The second golden era, stretching from the mid-1960s to the early 1980s, saw the development of a theoretical framework for epidemiology, clarification of concepts such as confounding and interaction and the emergence of case–control methodology. A brief description of the different types of epidemiology study is given in a later section.

There is no doubt that the post-World War II period has seen a tremendous upsurge in epidemiological activity and a parallel rise in concern over environmental and occupational health matters. The work of Doll and Hill (1950, 1954) was of great importance in demonstrating that cigarette smoking causes lung cancer, but it also established the methodology of case–control and cohort studies. However, the British doctors' cohort study reported by Doll and Hill (1954) was prospective and credit must also be given to the bladder cancer study by Case *et al.* (1954), which played a major role in establishing the credibility of the historical cohort study. Not only does the work Case stand up to scrutiny more than 30 years later, but also this study and the work of Cornfield (1951) on case–control studies have legitimized the use of retrospectively collected data and led to the historical cohort and case–control studies becoming the major techniques in modern cancer and mortality epidemiology.

The Framingham Heart Study initiated in 1949 to study risk factors for cardiovascular diseases was another major landmark in the development of epidemiology as a science. In addition to making a significant contribution to our understanding of the aetiology of cardiovascular disease, the Framingham study spurred the development of a large body of epidemiological methodology. However, despite the undoubted progress during the last 40 years, the science of epidemiology is still in its infancy. Rothman (1986) points to disagreements and confusion about the most basic concepts or measures leading to profound differences in the interpretation of data, and Feinstein (1988) notes that, depite peer review approval, current epidemiological methods need substantial improvement to produce trustworthy scientific evidence.

Epidemiological End-Points

The end-points studied by epidemiologists and toxicologists serve to illustrate some of the major differences between the two sciences. An excellent review of epidemiological end-points and their measurement is provided in a WHO publication on guidelines on studies in environmental epidemiology (World Health Organization, 1983). The end-points studied by epidemiologists and toxicologists are broadly similar–namely organ malfunction, death, carcinogenesis, birth defects and mutagenesis. However, only in the case of cancer is the epidemiologist likely to obtain the same quality of information about the end-point as is the toxicologist. An epidemiologist conducting a study of workers exposed to a heptotoxin will be reliant on haematology and clinical chemistry laboratory test results. The toxicologist will of course also make use of the same indicators of lier malfunction but will also have access to other measures of subacute or chronic toxicity such as the organ weight at neceropsy and histopathology. Even in the case of a discrete end-point such as death, the epidemiologists is reliant on death certificates for information. Many studies of the accuracy of death certificates have shown that the individual causes listed on the certificate are often identified incorrectly. The quality and limitations of death registration data are discussed in the decennial occupational mortality supplement of the Office of Population Censuses and Survey (OPCS) (1986), in England and Wales. It is noted there that the errors are generally greater for deaths of the elederly and for deaths from certain conditions, notbaly cerebrovascular disease. As an illustration, Doll and Peto (1981) argue that in recent years the old have received in creasingly careful medical attention, which must affect artefactually the trends in cancer death certification rates. Consequently they restricted a study of trends in cancer incidence to people under the age of 65.

The epidemiologist is not at a total disadvantage, for there are certain health responses that the toxicologist would find difficult to measure in experimental studies of animals. The neuro-behavioural tests for studies of Organic Solvent Syndrome are one such example (World Health Organization, 1985). Results in human studies cannot usually be replicated or explored in animal models, because we do not know how animals 'think' or 'feel'. However, the study of reproductive disorders typifies the difficulties that epidemiologists sometimes face in obtaining health response data. The toxicological approach to the study of reproductive effects is described and is a well-established feature of regulatory submissions for agrochemicals and pharmaceutical products. The epidemiologist has considerable difficulty in measuring the reproductive efficiency of couples. Male functional performance has been measured in some industry studies using semen collected from workforce volunteers (e.g., Dobbins, 1987), but such an approach would be unacceptable in occupational and environmental studies in many countries. Decreases libido and functional disorders may be revealed by questionnaries but the value of such an approach has yet to be proven. Questionnaries have also been used to estimate the occurrence of menstrual disorder in women and to measure the reproductive efficiency of couples (Levine *et al.,* 1980). Kallen (1988) comprehensively reviews the end-points studied in reproductive epidemiology and the methods for collecting and interpreting data on spontaneous abortion and malformations. However, fetal loss rates are extremely difficult to quantify and the event may not even be noticed by the woman herself in the first trimester.

Questionnaires have been described in the discussion of reproductive epidemiology and represent another major difference between toxicology and epidemiology. The use of symption questionnaires is widespread in epidemiology and makes it possible to compare symptom prevalence in groups of individuals exposed to different agents. In the case of respiratory and cardiovascular epidemiology, standardized questionnaires are an extremely important research tool and considerable efforts have been made to ensure their validity and reproducibility (e.g., Medical Research Council, 1976; Rose *et al.,* 1982). Questionnaires are also used to quantify a number of ill-defined conditions such as stress (Goldberg, 1972), Sick Building Symdrom (Finnegan *et al.,* 1984) and allergy to laboratory animals (Botham *et al.,* 1987). They also form an important component of the range of neurological examination methods and the techniques used in epidemiological studies for assessing neurotoxic effects.

Measurement of Exposure

Wegman and Eisen (1988) make the valid point that epidemiologists have placed much greater emphasis on the measure of response than on the measure of exposure. They claim that this is because most epidemiologists have been trained as physicians and are consequently more oriented towards measuring health outcomes. It is certainly true that a modern textbook of epidemiology such as Rothman (1986) says very little about what the epidemiologist should do with exposure assessments. However, this is probably as much a reflection of the historical paucity of quantitative exposure information as a reflection on the background of epidemiologists. Nevertheless, it is surprising how many epidemiological studies do not contain even a basic qualitative assessment of exposure. Almost half 24, do not even specify the pesticides to which applicators were potentially exposed. The contrast between epidemiology and toxicology is never more marked than in the area of estimation of dose response. Not only can the toxicologist carefully control the conditions of the exposure to the agent of interest, but also he can be sure that his animals have not come into contact with any other toxic agents. The industrial epidemiologist conducting the study of workers exposed to a heptotoxin described in the previous section will certainly have to control for alcohol intake and possibly for exposure to other hepatotoxins in the work and home environment. Nevertheless, it can be argued that epidemiology studies more accurately measure the effect on human health of 'real-life' exposures.

In occupational studies it is often necessary to assess exposure retrospectively. Few companies have either recorded or kept quantitative exposure data over even the working lifetimes of their current employees.

Most manufacturing processes change considerably over time, as do the exposures experienced by the workforce. In addition, the ingredients and chemical reactions may not be well documented and can greatly complete the characterization of exposure. Often the epidemiologist has to rely on anecdotal evidence and careful detective work by an industrial hygienist to construct a matrix of exposures by job title and time-period. Occasionally attempts are made to estimate past exposures by reconstructing redundant industrial processes. Ayer *et al.,* (1973) describe the reconstruction of a old granite shed to estimate dust levels. Even if quantitative exposure data are available, obtained by either static monitor or personal sampler, it will almost certainly have been collected to determine compliance with internal or external regulations. More emphasis is placed on recording the higher levels which occur after spillages and plant malfunction, and this may render the exposure data inappropriate for use to define normal exposures encountered in the jobs. It is to be hoped that, in future, epidemiologists and hygienists can develop sampling strategies that generate exposure data suitable for both compliance and epidemiological purposes.

If an exposure matrix has been constructed with quantitative estimates of the exposure in each job and time-period, then it is a simple matter to estimate cumulative exposure. It is a more difficult process when, as commonly, only a qualitative measure of exposure is available–e.g. high, medium and low. Even when exposure measurements are available, it may not be sensible to make an assumption that an exposure which occurred 20 years ago is equivalent to the same exposure yesterday. The use of average exposures may also be questionable, and peak exposures may be more relevant in the case of outcomes such as asthma and chronic brochitis. Noise is a good example of an exposure which must be carefully characterized and where the simple calculation of a cumulative exposure may be milseading. There is now evidence that hearing loss due to noise is dependent on the mount of hearing already lost because of ageing (Robinson, 1987). It is also important to distinguish between continuous, intermittent and impulse noise when investigating noise-induced hearing loss. A further factor which is often not considered is the use of personal protective equipment. For instance, in the studies of noise-induced hearing loss it is rare to see an attempt made to correct for the protection afforded by ear-plugs, hearingmuffs, etc.

Epidemiological Study Designs

This section provides a brief introduction to the most important types of studies conducted by epdimologists. It is an attempt to briefly described the principles of the major types of epidemiological studies in order to assist the toxicologist to understand the reporting of epidemiological studies and the assumptions made by epidemiologists. The next section of this chapter will discuss the similarities and differences between the methodologies of toxicology and epidemiology.

Cohort Studies

Historical Cohort Study

When the need arises to study the health status of a group of workers, there is often a large body of historical data which can be utilized. If sufficient information exists on individual exposed in the past to a potential workplace hazard, then it may be possible to undertake a retrospective cohort study. The historical data will have been collected for reasons which have nothing to do with epidemiology. Nevertheless, the availability of personnel records such as starters' and leavers' registers, payrolls, work rosters and individuals' career records has enabled many epidemiological studies to be conducted–in particular, mortality studies.

The principles of a historical cohort study can also be applied to follow a cohort of workers propsectively. This approach will be discussed further in the next subsection, although it should be emphasized that many historical data studies have a prospective element in so far as they are updated after a further period of follow-up. The discussion of historical cohort studies in this section will concentrate on mortality and cancer incidence studies. However, there is no reason why hearing loss, lung function or almost any measure of the health status of an individual should not be studied retrospectively if sufficient information is available.

Mortality and cancer incidence studies are unique among retrospective cohort studies in that they can be conducted using national cancer and mortality registers even if there has been no medical suveillance of the workforce. A historical cohort study also has the advantages of being cheaper and providing estimates of the potential hazards much earlier than a prospective study. However, historical cohort studies are beset by a variety of problems. Principal among these is the problem of determining which workers have been exposed and, if so, to what degree. In addition, it may be difficult to decide what is a appropriate comparison group. It should also be borne in mind that in epidemiology, unlike animal experimentation, random allocation is not possible and there is no control over the factors which may distort the effects of the exposure of interest, such as smoking and standard of living.

The principles of historical cohort studies as they apply within a large chemical company in the UK are described in the following subsections.

Cohort Definition and Follow-up Period

A variety of sources of information are used to identify workers exposed to a particular workplace hazards, to construct and occupational history and complete the collection of information necessary for tracing. It is essential that the cohort be well defined and that criteria for eligibility be strictly followed. This requires that a clear statement be made about membership of the cohort so that it is easy to decide whether an employee is a member or not. It is also important that the follow-up period be carefully defined. For instance, it is readily apparent that the follow up period should not start before exposure has occurred. Furthermore, it is uncommon for the health effect of interest to manifest itself immeiately after exposure, and allowance for an appropriate biological induction (or latency) period may need to be made when interpreting the data.

Tracing

In the UK the vital status (alive, dead, emigrated or untraced) and the causes of death of members of a cohort study are ascertained by use of the National Health Service Central Resigter (NHSCR) of the UK. In the authors' Company it is also possible to ascertain the vital status of a large proportion of cohort members by use of company mortality registers and personnel records. NHSCR provides assistance to a wide variety of medical research projects in the UK. In addition to ascertaining the status of an individual on a given date, NHSCR will also flag live individuals and notify the study manager when they die. Consequently, it is a relatively simple matter to update a mortality study after a further period of follow-up.

Comparison Subjects

The usual comparison group for many studies is the national population. However, it is known that there are marked regional differences in the mortality rates for many causes of death. Regional mortality rates exist in the UK (e.g. Gardner *et al.,* 1984) but have to be used with caution because they are based on small numbers of deaths and estimated population sizes. In some situations the local rates for certain causes may be highly influenced by the mortality of the workforce being studied. Furthermore, it is not always easy to decide what the most appropriate regional rate for comparison purposes is, as many employees may reside in a different region from that in which the plant is situated.

An alternative or additional approach is to establish a cohort of unexposed workers for comparison purposes. However, workers with very low exposures to the workplace hazard will often provide similar information. A good discussion of the issues is found in the proceedings of a conference entirely devoted to the subject.

Analysis and Interpretation

In a cohort study the first stage in the analysis consists of calculating the number of deaths expected during the follow-up period. In order to calculate the expected death for the cohort, the survival experience of the cohort is broken down into individual years of survival known as 'person years'. Each person-year is characterized by the age of the cohort member and the time-period when survival occurred and the sex of the cohort member. The person-years are then multiplied by age, sex and time-period specific mortality rates to obtain the expected number of deaths.

Thus, an SMR of 125 represents an excess mortality of 25 per cent. An SMR can be calculated for different causes of death and for subdivision of the person-years by factors such as level of exposure and time since first exposure.

Interpretation of cohort studies is not always straightforward, and there are a number of selection effects and biases that must be considered (Rothman, 1986). Cohort studies routinely report that the mortality of active workers is less than that of the population as a whole. It is not an unexpected finding, since workers usually have to undergo some sort of selection process to become or remain workers. Nertheless, this selection effect, known as the 'healthy worker' effect, can lead to considerable arguments over the interpretation of study results, particularly if the cancer mortality is a expected, but the all-cause mortality is much lower than expected. Wee (1986) gives an interesting historical account of attempts to understand the process of occupational selection. However, even an experimental science such as toxicology is not without a similar problem of interpretation, viz. The problem of distinguishing between the effects of age and treatment on tumour incidence (Peto *et al.,* 1980).

Proportional Mortality Study

There are often situations where one has no accurate data on composition of a cohort but does possess a set of death records (or cancer registrations). Under these circumstances a proportional mortality study may sometimes be substituted for a cohort study. In such a mortality study the proportions of deaths from a specific cause among the study deaths is compared with the proportion of deaths from that cause in a comparison population. The results of a proportional mortality study are expressed in an analogous way to those of the cohort study with follow-up. Corresponding to the observed deaths from a particular cause, it is possible to calculate an expected number of deaths based on mortality rates for that cause and all causes of death in a comparison group and the total number of deaths in the study.

Thus, a PMR of 125 for a particular cause of death represents a 25 per cent increase in the proportion of deaths due to that cause. A proportional mortality study has the advantage of avoiding the expensive and time-consuming establishment and tracing of a cohort, but the disadvantage of little or no exposure information.

Prospective Cohort Study

Prospective cohort studies are no different in principle from historical cohort studies in terms of scientific logic, the major differences being timing and methodology. The study starts with a group of apparently healthy individuals whose health and exposure is studied over a period of time. As it is possible to define in advance the information that is to be collected, prospective studies are theoretically more reliable than retrospective studies. However, long periods of observation may be required to obtain results.

Prospective cohort studies or longitudinal studies of continually changing health parameters such as lung function, hearing loss, blood bio-chemistry and haematological measurements pose different problems from those encountered in mortality and cancer incidence studies. The relationships between changes in the parameters of interest and exposure measurements have to be estimated and, if necessary, a comparison made of changes in the parameters between groups. These relationships may be extremely complicated, compounded by factors such as ageing, and difficult to estimate, as there may be relatively few measurement points. Furthermore, large errors of measurement in the variables may be present because of factors such as within-laboratory variation and temporal variation within individuals. Missing observations and withdrawals may also cause problems, particularly if they are dependent on the level an change of the parameter of interest. These problems may make it difficult to interpret and judge the validity of analytical conclusions. Nevertheless, prospective cohort studies provide the best means of measuring changes in health parameters and relating them to exposure.

Case–Control Study

In a case–control study two groups of individuals are selected for study, of which one has to the desease whose causation is to be studied (the cases) and the other does not (the controls). In the context of the chemical industry, the aim of a case–control study is to evaluate the relevance of past exposure to the development of a disease. This is done by obtaining an indirect estimate of the rate of occurrence of the disease in an exposed and unexposed group by comparing the frequency of exposure among cases and controls.

Principal Features

Case–control and cohort studies complement each other as types of epidemiological study. In a case-control study the groups are defined on the basis of the presence or absence of a given disease and, hence, only one disease can be studied at a time. The case–control study compensates for this by providing information on a wide range of exposures which may play a role in the development of the disease. In controast, a cohort study generally focuses on a single exposure but can be analysed for multiple disease outcomes. A case–control study is a better way of studying rare diseases because a very large cohort would be required to demonstrate an excess of a rare disease. In contrast, a case–control study is an inefficient way of assessing the effect of an uncommon exposure, when it might be possible to conduct a cohort study of all those exposed. The complementary strengths and weakness of case–control and cohort studies can be used to advantage. Increasingly, mortality studies are being reported which utilize 'nested' case–control studies to investigate the association between the exposures of interest and a cause of death for which an excess has been discovered. However, case–control studies have traditionally been held in low regard, largely because they are often badly conducted and interpreted. There is also a tendency to overinterpret the data and misuse statistical procedures. In addition, there is still considerable debate among leading epidemiologists themselves as to how controls should be selected—e.g., Poole, (1986) and Schlesselman and Stadel (1987).

Analysis and Interpretation

In a case–control study it is possible to compare the frequencies of exposures in the cases and controls. However, what one is realy interested in is a comparison of the frequencies of disease in the exposed and the unexposed.

Matching

Matching is the selection of a comparison group that is, within stated limits, identical with the study group with respect to one or more factors such as age, years of service, smoking history, etc., which may distort the effect of the exposure of interest. The matching may be done on an individual or group basis. Although matching may be used in all types of study, including follow-up and cross-sectional studies, it is more widely used in case–control studies. It is common to see case–control studies in which each case is matched to as many as three or four controls.

Nested Case–Control Study

In a cohort the assessment of exposure for all cohort members may be extremely time-consuming and demanding of resources. If an excess of death or incidence has been discovered for a small number of conditions, it may be much more efficient to conduct a case–control study in to investigate the effect of exposure. Thus, instead of all members being studied, only the cases and a sample of non-cases would be compared with regard to exposure history. Thus, there is no need to investigate the exposure histories of all those who are neither cases nor controls. However, the nesting is only effective if there are a reasonable number of cases and sufficient variation in the exposure of the cohort members.

Other Study Designs

Descriptive Studies

There are large numbers of records in existence which document the health of various groups of people. Mortality statistics are available for many countries and even for certain companies. Similarly, there is a wide range of routine morbidity statistics—in particular, those based on cancer registrations. These health statistics can be used to study differences between geographic regions (e.g. maps of cancer mortality and incidence presented at a recent Symposium, Boyle *et al.,* 1989), occupational groups and time periods. Investigations based on existing records of the distribution of disease and of possible causes are known as descriptive studies. It is sometimes possible to identify hazards associated with the development of rare conditions from observation of clustering in occupational or geographical areas. The report by Creech and Johnson (1974) on 3 cases of haemangiosarcoma in vinyl chloride workers at the B.F. Goodrich Chemical Company is a good example. At that time only 25 cases a year of haemanigosarcoma were reported for the whole of the United States. However, much more detailed information on the population at risk and valid comparison rates are usually required to allow sensible interpretation of mortality and morbidity statistics.

Cross-sectional Study

Cross-sectional studies measure the cause (exposure) and the effect (disease) at the same point in time. They compare the rates of diseases or symptoms of an exposed group with an unexposed group. Strictly speaking, the exposure information is ascertained simultaneously with the disease information. In practice, such studies are usually more meaningful from an aetiological or causal point of view if the exposure assessment reflects past exposures. Current information is often all that is available but may still be meaningful, because of the correlation between current exposure and relevant past exposure.

Cross-sectional studies are widely used to study the health of groups of workers who are exposed to possible hazards but do not undergo regular surveillance. They are particularly suited to the study of subclinical parameters such as blood bio-chemistry and haematological values. Cross-sectional studies are also relatively straightforward to conduct in comparison with prospective cohort studies and are generally simpler to interpret.

Intervention Study

Not all epidemiology is observational, and experimental studies have a role to play in evaluating the efficiency of an intervention programme to prevent disease–e.g. fluoridation of water. An intervention study at one extreme may closely resemble a clinical trial with individuals randomly selected to receive some form of intervention–e.g. advice on reducing cholesterol levels. However, in some instances it may be a whole community that is selected to form the intervention group. The selection may or may not be random. The toxiclogist might argue that even if selection was random, such a study of two communities, each consisting of many individuals, was in a sense a study of only two subjects. However, he should ask himself first whether the 'three rats to a cage' design of many subacute toxicity studies really generates three independent responses per cage.

The Epidemiology Toxicology Interface

Beginning in the early 1990s the protection of human health from chemicals in the workplace, market place and environment has become a universally recognized goal. The approach towards this goal has developed over time and can be roughly characterized by three processes (Friess, 1987): (1) the development of some form of human dose-response relationship for an adverse health effect; (2) the assessment of risk for that effect under specific exposure conditions; and (3) the setting of permissible exposure limits for the chemical in various exposure scenarios. At the beginning of the twentieth century the US government passed the first Food and Drug Act, aimed at regulating the widespread adulteration of food with chemical additives. To identify some chemicals and to emphasize the problems, Dr. Harvey Wiley conducted the first toxicology studies for regulatory purposes on behalf of the Bureau of Chemistry (which subsequently became the Food and Drug Administration) by setting up feeding experiments with 12 healthy, male volunteers (Glocklin, 1987). It soon became apparent that there were insidious, even lifethreatening, toxicities, lurking in foodstuffs and patent medicines which went far beyond the transient gastroinstinal upsets or general malaise that Dr. Wiley's so-called 'poison squad' would have been willing to accept. The ethical concerns with human studies quickly led to the use of animals in safety testing.

By developing strains of laboratory animals and maintaining them in good health and in a controlled environment, it was possible to carry out reproducible experiments, and the science of experimental toxicology came into existence (Zapp, 1981). However, ever since toxicologists came to rely on surrogate models for man, arguments about trans-species prediction in assessing human health hazards have been a major issue (Brown and Paddle, 1988).

Methodological Differences

The interface between epidemiology and toxicology is sometimes fraught. The toxicologist argues that the tighter specification of animal studies, and the absence of the social and environmental factors which confuse the issue in human studies, should lead one to regard the animal studies as more informative. However, the epidemiologist would counter that the greater relevance of the species, and the greater relevance of the dose in that species, make the epidemiological data more informative.

The toxicologist will have noticed certain similarities between the prospective cohort study and the carcinogenesis bioassay and other approaches to chronic toxicity testing. The use of national mortality statistics for comparison purposes may seem odd to the toxicologist but is analogous to the use of historical information in toxicology studies. The most obvious difference, however, is the inability of the epidemiologist randomly to assign workers to the different exposure groups. Randomization does play a part in epidemiology, as can be seen in the description of intervention studies. The cross-sectional study will also be recognized by the toxicologist as being the analogue of a subacute toxicity study. Although many of the study endpoints are similar (e.g. haematology and clinical chemistry test results), the epidemiologist will also study a much larger range of health effects such as respiratory function (lung function testing and X-ray changes) and blood pressure. However, unlike the toxicologists, the epidemiologist is unable to look for histopathological changes in the tissues of subjects. The studies that will seem most alien to the toxicologist are the retrospective studies. They clearly have no counterpart in toxicology or any other experimental science, although it is interesting to note that Schlesselman (1982) claims that the case-control approach was formalized within the field of sociology during the 1920s.

The differences become most apparent when one considers carcinogens. It is both unethical and impractical to expose humans to compounds and wait and see (typically 15–30 years) whether cancers result. Animal studies are not so constrained by either ethics or time. A rodent bioassay can be completed within 3 years (animal life-span = 2 years; pathological and quantitative analyses up to 1 year) and therefore toxicology may be described as a prospective study, while epdemilogy is largely retrospective. The poorer quality of some epidemiological end-points, particularly those based on death certification, has already been discussed. The epidemiologist has little control over the health of subjects on entry but, as noted previously, the health of an employee at recruitment is likely to be better than average. However, the health of a subject at recruitment will be one factor that influences the response of the subject to exposure to the agent under study. In addition, there may be many other confounding factors such as age, smoking habits, alcohol consumption, diet and exposure to other hazards at work and at home. By comparison, the toxicologist can be confident of minimal confounding effects and pure compound exposure, and has the reassurance provided by his trail control data of detecting genuine compound-related effects.

A further difference between the two types of study is in the pattern and level of exposure. Both animal and human studies may be investigating the same chemical but the means to the end is quite different. Suppose that the compound of interest is a pesticide used in spraying corn maize. Then two potential human groups to study would be: (1) applicators, having exposure seasonally to significant amounts, then periods of no exposure at all (i.e. pulse doses), and possibly concurrent exposure to other chemicals; and (2) the general population, who may consume the product on average twice a week in only very small amounts as a food contaminant. Not only is the pattern and level of exposure different for the two groups of humans potentially at risk, but also the routes of exposure are dissimilar. The applicators are exposed by skin absorption, inhalation and oral routes to more than one pesticide, while the general population is exposed by the oral route. The toxicology study, however, would be conducted as a 7 days a week, lifetime feeding study with the only control variable being the single pesticide of interest. Dose levels would be defined around the maximum tolerance dose (MTD), and some subfraction thereof.

These three different exposure scenarios–(1) human, 'pulse dose' to more than one chemical; (2) human, intermittent very low doses and (3) animal, constant high levels–exemplify how exposure patterns, levels and routes can vary not only within a species, but also between species. Epidemiogists of necessity study populations of great genetic heterogeneity and of wide age distribution (at least within 16–65 years for industrial working age range and lifetime years for environmental agents). They are populations exposed intermittently to largely unknown concentrations of the toxicant of interest, by an ill-defined combination of routes, almost never in isolation, for outcomes or effects which are rarely determinable or even definable in the precise terms which are demanded of animal studies (Utidjian, 1987).

Species Differences

There are a number of biological factors which may enhance the susceptibility to an individual to experience adverse health effects from exposure to toxic substances. The include age, sex, genetic composition, nutritional status and pre-existing disease conditions (Calabrese, 1986). The extent or magnitude to which predisposing factors enhance susceptibility to toxic substances is known only to a limited extent. The conversion of estimated risks from animal studies conducted at high doses to estimated risks for human at lower doses involves several considerations: (1) scaling for differences in size, life-span, metabolic rate (*quantitative differences*); (2) adjustment for differences in route of exposure or absorption (*qualitative differences*); (3) adjustment for bio-chemical and pharmacokientic differences (*qualitative and quantitative differences*); (4) consideration of interspecies differences in inherent susceptibility (*qualitative differences*). These four considerations can be grossly divided between quantitative and qualitative differences. Considerations (2), (3) and (4) are considered to be qualitative, as generally the pharmacokinetics, pharmacodynamics and mechanisms of action for individual toxins in a variety of species by different routes have many data gaps.

In terms of dose comparisons between animal studies and man, the quantitative differences assume greater importance over the qualitative differences because the database is more complete. The preferred scaling factor involves relating the dose to the species surface area, since this allometric relationship is a reflection of basal metabolic rate. Trans-species comparison to toxicity have shown that surface area scaling provides the best correlation, and consequently this approach has been adopted by the EPA (US EPA, 1980).

The allometric relationship between toxicity and species surface area may indeed provide an adequate, if not refined, method for cross-species predictivity. However, the literature is scattered with examples that reveal either marked underestimation or overestimation of the risks for man. Formaldehyde is an example where risk assessments based on animal data have overestimated the risks for man. The dose levels at which animal tumours were observed (Kerns *et al.,* 1983) resulted in overestimation of the risks for man (US EPA, 1987), which directly conflict with several epidemiology studies (Acheson *et al.*, 1984; Blair *et al.*, 1986). On the other hand, there are examples where epidemiology has revealed toxic effects in man at far lower levels than the animal models would predict–e.g. vinyl chloride (Purchase, 1985) and benzene (Wong, 1987). Indeed there are several reviews which address the relative species sensitivity to specific carcinogens (Anderson and Campbell, 1985); Williams *et al.*, 1985; dybing, 1986 Gregory, 1988), and it would appear that these conflicts (Purchase 1980a, 1985; Brown and Paddle, 1988) are due not to quantitative differences but to metabolic or mechanistic qualitative species differences. It might then be appropriate to suggest that more metabolic and biochemically orientated investigations in species differences could result in a greater understanding of the frequent anomalies between toxicology and epidemiology study results.

Site Concordance and Predictability

Sir Richard Doll has noted that most recognized occupational cancers have been discovered as a result of clinical intuition or epidemiological observation. However, most could have been avoided if modern toxicological techniques had been employed to test the substances used before humans were exposed to them in the industrial environment (Doll, 1984). Virtually all of the chemicals that have been demonstrated to the causative agents of cancer in humans also produce cancer in a variety of animal models (Henschler, 1987). On the basis of this substantial background of evidence that human carcinogens can be revealed in animal models, it has been widely assumed that chemicals that are carcinogenic in animal models are likely to be potential cancer hazards to man. This assumption has been reinforced by instances in which chemicals have been demonstrated to be carcinogenic in animals before subsequent identification of cancer causation in humans; examples of this are vinyl chloride (Maltoni, 1977) and bis(chloromethyl) ether.

Doll (1981) commented on the agreement between

carcinogenicity testing results in rats and mice for 250 chemicals reported by Purchase (1980b). The agreement between rats and mice for 83 per cent of compounds is ubstantially higher than would be expected by chance (50 per cent). Henschler (1987) concluded that 96 per cent of the 56 occupational cacinogens in the 1984 German MAK list were predictable by animal experiments. The only two compounds that were given as possible errors in predictability were arsenicals and benzene. It would be very comforting indeed to feel that toxicology provides such an adequate safety testing system/network to avoid epidemiologically discovered errors. However, one cannot judge a screening test in terms of its sensitive alone. The International Agency for Research on Cancer (IARC, 1987) classified 50 chemicals and industrial processes as human carcinogens, and of these there was sufficient evidence to classify 21 as carcinogenic to both humans and experimental animals. However, many of these agents produce tumours at several sites and there is agreement in respect of only one site. Nevertheless, compounds for which tumours are induced in the animals but at sites not in accordance with the human data can generally be reasoned by virtue of differential metabolism–e.g., benzidine and 2-naphthylamine. It is apparent that human carcinogens are generally characterized by overt genetic toxicity (Shelby, 1988) and that tumour induction for genotoxins is ubiquitous trans-species.

Although it may be possible to examine the sensitivity of experimental testing in animals as an indicator of carcnogenicity in humans, it is extremely difficult to examine is specificity. IARC (1987) classify only one chemical. Other agents are classified as having evidence suggesting lack of carcinogenicity in experimental animals, but no agent (including caprolactam) is classified as such in terms of human carcinogenicity. Thus we cannot estimate how many times animal testing wrongly predicts carcinogenicity in humans.

Summary

Utidjian (1987) provides for several compounds a comprehensive review of the ways in which epidemiology has historically interacted with animal toxicity studies. Utidjian concludes that epidemiology has started to lose its historic role as the initiating or hypothesis-generating discipline and has become a secondary tool to confirm, refute or quantify human carcinogenic effects, the animal carcnogenesis bioassay being responsible for this change in role. This is undoubtedly true to some degree, and Utidjian cites acrylonitrile, formaldehyde, ethylene oxide and acrylamide as examples where the results of animal carcinogenesis bioassays have triggered a flurry of epidemiology studies. However, cancer is not the only health effect of interest to medical investigators and regulators. For instance, Axelson *et al.,* (1976) first described the syndrome now known as Organic Solvent Syndrome or 'Danish painters' disease' and a tentative association between the syndrome and chronic exposure to solvents. The report not led to much epidemiological work, but also stimulated toxicologists to take a greater interest in neurobehavioural effects. Even in the case of carcinogenesis, the increasing interest taken by IARC in occupations and mixtures is likely to strengthen the hand of epidemiology. It is clear in the case of nicely and chromium that epidemiological evidence first indicated that certain nickel and chromium compounds must be carcinogens. However, the early studies led to much speculation as to what the specific carinogens. However, the early studies led to much speculation as to what the specific carcinogenic agent or agents might be. Animal studies were conducted in an attempt to elucidate the situation, and the combination of evidence from the two disciplines has led to the identification of certain chromium compounds a human carcinogens, although the nickel debate continues. Epidemiology will undoubtedly continue to point the first finger of suspicion at occupations or processes that involve a mixture of compounds. The case–control study has an important role to play as a hypothesis generator and is a particularly potent research tool in the Scandinavian countreis, where there exist compouterized record systems linking census information and health data.

There can be little doubt that the relationship between epidemiology and toxicology should be an interaction. Although the two disciplines are methodologically very different and sometimes generate conflicting results, they should be seen as complementary. In this chapter we have tried to describe the strenghs and weaknesses of each discipline and to indicate the need for co-operation between epidemiologists and toxicologists. Both share a common goal–human health protection. Toxicology in essence is animal epidemiology, and epidemiology can be viewed as an opportunistic analysis of the inadvertent exposure of humans to toxicants. Kamrin (1988) goes further when describing the different types of toxicity testing, and includes epidemiology as the fourth major study design alongside acute toxicity testing, subacute toxicity testing and chronic toxicity testing in animal experiments. The toxicologist must be prepared to recognize the greater relevance of epidemiology to assessing risks to humans, but the epidemiologist must also be prepared to acknowledge the high degree of site concordance (for overt genotoxins) and the additional number of non-concordants (but with carcinogenic activity) of the 50 known human carcinogens. Sir Richard Doll (1981), in an article on the relevance of epidemiology to policies for the prevention of cancer, concluded that '... no rational person would want to learn by counting dead bods if he could possibly learn by other means how their particular causes of death could have been avoided' and 'Epidemiology may not be the method of choice for the discovery of preventative measures, as it requires some people to have been affected before it can be employed; but at present its use is essentia....' These remarks clearly indicate the need for both toxicologists and epidemiologists to be aware of the contributions their respective disciplines can make in assecing human health hazards.

3

Pharmaceutical Toxicology

It is salutary to look back in recent time and realize that the Committee on Safety of Drugs (the Dunlop Committee), which was established on a voluntary basis in the UK in 1963, was not directly concenred with drug efficacy. The voluntary arrangements were dominated by safety; the Committee's remit did not impose upon it any responsibility to consider the efficiacy of drugs except insofar as their safety was concerned. It is only since 1971 that an integrated regulatory system concerned with all the three requriements–safety, efficancy and quality of medicinal products–was introduced into the UK through the implementation of the Medicines Act of 1968.

This enactment placed special empahsis on considerations of safety in relation to the issue of both Product Licences and ceinical Trials Certificats (Section 36.2). In contrast with its provisions in respect of efficacy, the Medicines Act allowed the Licensing Authority to take account of comparative safety in deciding applications. Moreover, the Act took a broad view of safety by including not only potential dangers to patients themselves, but also hazards to the community and to those administering the drugs; it also covered interference with diagnosis; treatment or prevention of disease. Comparable requirements within the European Community are contained in the relevant

EEC Directives (Commission of the European Communities, 1984). Matters which have potential financial implications, such as clinical need and comparative efficacy, are specifically excluded from both the Medicins Act in the UK and the EEC Directives.

In attempting to ensure the safety of drugs the Licensing Authority and the Committee on safety of Medicines in the UK rely on three strategies–the control of quality, reigorous pre-marketing safety studies and post-marketing surveillance. Quality is controlled in relat-ion to both manufacture and wholesale selling and, as a consequence, toxicity due to product defects is now exceptional (Rawlings, 1989).

There are no priorities within safety, quality and efficancy, for all three requirements are equally wighted. Default in any one will jeopardize marketing approval or continuation of clinical use. Stephens (1988) summed up the situation thus: '... in future it will no longer be sufficient for pharmaceutical companies to plan their clinical trial programme for a new drug on the basis of showing that it is efficacious (ADRs) were noted. The cost half of the cost/benefit ratio now demands that equal effort must be put into active research for adverse reactions as in the proof for efficacy.' Thus, the evaluation of the toxic potential of a new molecule must be an active search, not merely a passive observation of what toxicity emerges during preliminary studies and subsequent clinical use.

Responsibility

The discovery of the ADR profile of a new drug prior to marketing lies entirely within the sphere of the pharmaceutical company and, therefore, the company has the responsibility for providing adquate information. After a drug is marketed, the responsibility for extending the knowledge base of its adverse reactions spreads also to all the prescribers of that drug, as well as to specific organizations set up for that purpose.

The predominant objective of all national and international drug regulations is to ensure the safety of marketed medicinal products during normal conditions of use. It could be defined as protecting the public health and safeguarding the public purse, for such prcedures also ensure that the patient gets value for money spent on the medication.

Drug Disasters
(Pre- and Post thalidomide)

Modern drug regulation in the UK was conceived in the aftermath of the thalidomide disaster. There is evidence that earlier disasters were equally troublesome, although perhaps not so well publicized as thalidomide. There have also been other disasters before and since thalidomide.

For example, jaundice and hepatic necrosis ('yellow atrophy of the liver') reached epidemic levels following the use of organo-arsenicals such as slavarsan to treat syphilis in soldiers returning from World War I.

Amidopyrine was commonly used as an antipyrctic and analgestic and it took almost half a century of common use to recognize that if caused agranulocytosis.

The ill-fated Elixir of Sulfanilamide produced by the old established Massengil Company in the United States not only heralded the new era of the sulphonamide drugs, but also during September and October 1937 directly caused at least 76 deaths due to the renal toxicity of its 72 per cent content of the solvent diethylene glycol; many of the victims were children. The sulphanilamide disaster shocked the country and was instrumental in Congress reacting by passing the Food, Drug and Cosmetic Act in 1938, which required all new drugs to be demonstrated to be safe.

Stalinon, a preparation designed to treat boils, led to a two-year prison sentence for its French inventor; it contained diiodoethyla tin and isoloinoleic acid esters and was associated with raised intracranial pressure. The product was alleged to have killed 102 people and permanently affected 100 more, some survivors having residual paraplegia.

Phenacetin was first used in 1887 and is an effective analgesic and antipyretic; unfortunately, however, it also has a long and somewhat controversial association with chronic renal disease, especially in the Swedish town of Huskvana, where local custom among the munition workers involved the frank abuse of Hjorton's Powders, which contained caffeine, phenacetin and phenazone.

The thalidomide tragedy is well known, as also is the SMON (subacute myelo-opticoneuropathy) epidemic in Japan due to the use of clioquinol for enteric disroders; both have received much publicity and were directly responsible for a greater awareness of the public of adverse drug reactions and a demand through their legislators for stricter controls over medicines.

Practolol, a very useful member and foreunner of the beta-blockers, gave rise to oculomucocutaneous syndrome and was withdrawn from general use.

Metamizol (novaminsulfon), a non-steroidal anti-anflammatory agent, was associated with blood dyscrasias.

The hypnotic agent triazolam, a benzodiazepine derivative, was associated with excitation reactions and acute psychic derangement: reactions that were complicated in 1979 by media induced suggestion and excitement in the Netherlands–the 'so-called' Halcion story. The Licensing Authority withdrew this medicine from the UK market in October 1991; an appeal is in progress.

Osmosin is worthy of particular mention because it was the formulation and not its indomethacin content that was the problem. This ustained-action (release) formulation 'dumped' its contents into the gut, causing ulceration and fatal intestinal perforation.

The non-steroidal anti-inflammatory agents (NSAIDs) have been singularly unfortunate in their marketing history. Benoxaprofen caused fatal hepatic reactions in the elderly patient and photosensitivity and onycholysis on a massive scale. It had a very short market life and it well illustrated the suddeness with which a true epidemic of adverse events can occur. Zomepirac another NSAID, was withdrawn because of the large numbers of incidents of serious anaphylaxis and allergic reactions that were associated with its use, while fenclofenac was withdrawn from the UK market in 1984, owing to a cluster of ADRs, including skin rashes, gastrointestinal disorders and suspected carcinogenicity. In the same year feprozone was withdrawn because of associated skin rashes, gastrointestinal disorders, thrombocytopenia, and haemolytic anaemia. Other problems with marketed drug products have followed in succeeding years.

The thalidomide tragedy looms so ponderously over the history of adverse drug reactions that it causes other events that have since occurred to pale into insignificance and even suggests that since 1961 the worst of the problems have been solves. This is just not so! The number of patients gravely injured or killed in epidemics of drug induced disease since then is a vast multiple of the number of thalidomide victims. Although much information has been gained about the circumstances leading to these individual disasters, there is little in these collections of data that will serve to prevent other drug disasters occurring that are qualitatively different from those that have gone before. The range of injuries produced is so wide that no single solution to the detection of future drug-induced disasters before they occur seems likely to emerge.

Regulations Concerned With Safety

Pharmaceutical toxicology is quite a different field from industrial or pesticide toxicity evaluations. The techniques employed and the methodology used are similar but the orientation is different. Since there is no way to providing the complete safety of a new drug before it comes into widespread use, it becomes a question of at what stage of development the risks should be defined. The easy answer is: as soon as possible, so that as few patients as possible are exposed to unnecessary risks. The regulatory authority must therefore weigh the advantages of the efficacy of a new drug, compared with the normal prognosis of the disease with known therapy, against the risks involved in marketing the new drug without full knowledge of its adverse reaction burden. At the same time the regulatory authority has to decide whether to leave the detection of the more rare side-effects to be discovered by the present testing systems or whether they should institute a major surveillance programme so that these risks may be known earlier.

The regulation of medicines by society has been expressed by Lasagna (1989) as being time-bound, country-bound and person-bound. It is time-bound both because of what are thought to be socially necessary changes over the years and because the sciences of medicine and pharmacology are constantly evolving. It is country-bound because each nation, in setting up its own regulatory system, will be guided by the particular needs of its citizens for medicines, its economy its political philosophy and the quality and extent of its scientific establishment and its health care delivery system. It is person-bound because no matter what the letter of the law may be for regulating medicines, or the nature of the published regulations, there is always the opportunity for value judgements to be made by those implementing the laws and regulations.

In considering the role of regulation, it is useful to be realistic about what can and what cannot be achieved by regulations, even when based on scientific rules of evidence and on accepted approaches to decision making. Traditionally, the most ancient and in a sense the least controversial function of regulation has been to ensure that a medicine is accurately labelled as to its contents, and the nature of the ingredients and their amounts (Lasagna, 1989). It is more difficult, however, to delineate the safety and efficacy of the medicine proposed for registration. Since the ability to explore the full dose–response curve for a drug's toxicity is not ethically possible in humans, it is necessary to rely to a great extent on animal studies to achieve insights into this relationship.

The Use of Animals in Safety Testing

There are powerful scientific, ethical and regulatory

reasons for exploring the effect of potential therapeutic candidates in animals before they are administered to man. There are also strong and public emotive reaons why they should not be used. However, the low proportion of significant toxic reactions in humans with new medicines, compared with the number tested and introduced, supports the contention that toxicity studies in laboratory animals are, in the main, predictive for man. There are also many positive occurrences between the findings in animal toxicity tests and adverse reactions in humans, particularly for dose- and time-related toxic effects. On the contrary, there have been well publicized accounts of failures of experimental toxicology and false alramrs resulting from apparently irrelevant toxicological observations in animals. The overall success of the current preclinical safety evaluation process is difficult to assess. Although useful information could be obtained by retrospective analysis of data obtained fro compounds that have been used extensively in the clinic, to date this has received only limited systematic study (Lumley and Walker, 1990).

In 1989, the Sixth Centre for Medicines Research (CMR), held in the Ciba Foundation in London, provided the opportunity for an international group of experts from the pharamcetutical industy, academia and the regulatory authorities to review critically and dicuss past methodologies which have been employed to assess the efficacy of animal toxicity testing procedures in predicting qualitative toxicity in man. Conventional animal toxicological stuies have three purposes: they attempt to define a compound's general toxicological profile; they are expected to reveal those target organs/systems demanding special study during clinical trails; and, it is hoped, they will provide a basis for predicting human safety (Rawlings, 1989). A most important aspect of the correlation of toxic effects between man and animals is the selection of animal species in which the drug is absorbed, distributed, metabolized and exreted in a similar manner to man.

The value of multispecies toxicity studies and parallel

metabolic studies has been well established (Morton, 1990). Yet despite wide experience with animal studies, their validity remains uncertain (Zbinden, 1981). Only a few investigators (Fletcher, 1978; Griffin, 1983; Laurence *et al.*, 1984) have attempted to correlate findings during human use with those observed during preclincial toxicity studies, and even these have been limited in scale and scope (Rawlings, 1989). Routine animal toxicity tests are most useful when there are no important qualitative differences between species and where one can make up for the difficulty in demonstrating certain adverse effects with clinically relevant doses in animals by administering the drug at very high doses, on the assumption that more sensitive individuals will respond in similar fashion when given smaller doses of the drug (Lasagna, 1989).

Carcinogenicity and Mutagenicity Testing

Unfortunately, there is current reliance on carcinogenicity and mutagenicity tests whose power and reliability are in question. Morton (1990) has summarized problems with the evaluation of animal mutagenicity and carcinogencity tests and their prediction of potential carcinogenicity in humans.

For many years potential new drugs have been tested at high doses in long-term carcinogenicity studies in rodents prior to regulatory approval and broad clinical use. These studies have been costly in test chemicals, animals, laboratory facilities and staff, and research time. Although the overall database on animal bioassays has been greatly expanded by the United States National Cancer Institute and the National Toxicology Programme, the prediction of human carcinogenicity is still problematic. In many studies the results have varied between species, strains and sexes of the animals tested. The incidence of tumours observed has not always been dose-related and the relevance of these studies to human carcinogenesis is still not clear.

Short-term mutagenicity tests are expected to detect genotoxic carcinogens, and a strong rationale has been developed for the use of these tests early in the process of drug development. Although neither a positive nor a negative result in short-term teests can be considered fully definitive, the International Agency for Research on Cancer has noted that the majority of chemicals that have given sufficient evidence of inducing human tumours are genotoxic (International Agency for Research on Cancer, 1987).

During recent years, however, it has become evident that the early estimates of the predictability of the mutagenicity tests for the carcinogenic properties of most chemicals were too optigenic properties of most chemicals were too optimistic (Shelby and Stasiewicz, 1984; Tennant *et al.,* 1987). A careful validation of *in vitro* tests against the results of long-term rodent carcinogenicity tests by Tennant *et al.,* (1987) found that none of the short-term tests were necessarily predictive. In fact, it was suggested that no combination of the available *in vitro* mutagenicity tests (e.g. Ames bacterial mutation; L5178Y mammalian mutation; rat hepatocyte DNA repair; CHO cell cytogenetics) was significantly better than a single test. Furthermore, Clayson (1987) has suggested that short-term tests cannot be expected to detect all types of carcinogens, since mutations may only be related to the initiation phase of the complex process of carcinogenesis. Further evidence has been given by Morton (1990), who has described and quoted mutagenicity testing in the laboratories of Eli Lilly and Company; in these validation studies most of the known human or animal carcinogens were detected in the broadly used and well-accepted batterly of *in vitro* and *in vivo* mutagenicity tests. However, when research compounds were tested in this tier, the number of positive findings was relatively small and in no case did a compound produce a positive response in more than one test.

Translation of Results from Animals to Man

When one moves from animals to humans, a conservative approach is usually taken, starting with doses in healthy volunteers at only a fraction of those which produce significant toxicity in the most sensitive animal species. It is generally agreed that in these earliest human studies, and in the subsequent clinical trails in Phases I and II, one can gain considerable insight into those adverse reactions that occur with some frequency. However, it is usually not possible to detect in the studies the truly rare serious side-effect, to say nothing of the side-effect that is long delayed in its onset, or occurs as a result of an interaction with basic diseases processes, or with other drugs. All that will eventually be known about the drug's effects, both good an bad, will never be known at the time of initial marketing of a compound. The lesson is obvious: efficient and skilful post registration observations must be relied upon to identify and prove cause–effect relationships between the taking of a drug and the occurrence of an untoward event.

Prospective studies designed to assess the relevance and predictive value of animal toxicity studies for man are rarely possible for ethical reasons (Brimblecombe, 1990). Substances showing marked toxicity in animals can only rarely, for ethical reasons, be administered to man. Prospective studies are, therefore, only possible with subtances showing an acceptable toxicological profile in animals. In general, there is a paucity of data in this area. However, although retrospective collection and analysis of data are less satisfactory, they are none the less important alternatives. Such data are available, for example, within pharmaceutical companies, but analysis of larger database such as those in regulatory authorities or those collected from a number of companies (for example, by the Centre for Medicines Research) has the potential for yielding more valuable information. Brimblecombe (1990) has suggested that retrospective studies can take a number of forms:

(1) Re-evaluation of data from animal studies when unwanted effects occur subsequently and unexpectedly in man.
(2) Design of specific animal studies to elucidate mechanisms of unwanted effects which have been

observed in man.

(3) Pooling of data from a number of sources to increase the size of the database and to enable more meaningful 'epidemiological-type' analyses to be performed.

(4) Reviews of the history of individual compounds which have been, or are in, development.

Bass (190), in summarizing the toxicologist's viewpoint on what could be learned by examining the data in the files of regulatory authorities, stated that data in those files highlighted the problem areas that exist in extrapolating the results of animal studies to man. Since animal toxicity studies should be performed for the sake of man, this implies differences for each developmental product; thus, it is no longer appropriate to work to generalized and rigid guidelines. Flexibility in itself seems insufficient if the pharmaceutical manufacturer does not know how the regulatory authorities will react to the test programmes envisaged, and if revision through interaction with the clinical level is not included. Bass concluded that the question to be answered is not whether studies available retrospectively have been of relevance to man and to what extent or percentage, but how to make such studies useful and relevant in the future. Thus, early interaction between the pharmaceutical manufacturer and the regulatory authority may be needed case by case. This, he believes, should reduce the overall number of toxicological studies, rendering those remaining as requirements more relevant.

Fletcher (1990), expressing the clinician's viewpoint, commented on the number of guidelines that have been introduced since 1977 which were similar but not identical: the toxicology guidelines of the Committee for Proprietary Medicinal Products (CPMP); the OECD toxicity testing guidelines; the Annexes of the Sixth Amendment Directive of the EEC, which were also toxicological guidelines; and the Guidelines for Good Laboratory Practice. The problem with these is that they have codified and ritualized toxicity testing, so that there is very little flexibility. In his view this was not ideal, for what was needed was a possibility of matching toxicological requirements to particular compounds.

There is a great deal of potential in examining the files of regulatory authorities, as these have a unique value in that they cover a whole range of compounds and therapeutic classes, providing the full range of toxicological and clinical testing. However, access to data held by regulatory authorities is strictly limited, since any one company has access only to information on its own compounds and the only place in which the totality exists is with the regulatory authorities. Fletcher (1990) has suggested how the situation could be improved. First, the inclusion of toxico-kinetics in current safety evaluation studies would provide the opportunity to compare pharmaco-kinetics and metabolism in animals with man and could prevent inappropriate conclusions being drawn with regard to animal and human conditions. Second, there is an urgent need for closer co-operation between toxicologists and clinicians in the industry. Finally, detailed analyses of toxicological and clinical data available from regulatory authorities should be carried out.

Fletcher (1990) has suggested that this could be approached by tabulating and analysing all the anatomical, physiological and toxicological findings for particular groups of chemically or therapeutically similar compounds. This would give insight into whether they are consistent or inconsistent and what could and could not be relied upon. He also suggested an analysis of time relationships to identify situations that have proved to be consistently unreliable, inappropriate or irrelevant. This should provide evidence as to whether long-term tests—for example, in dogs–were irrelevant.

Lumley (1990) has provided interesting information on the termination of development by companies as a result of clinical toxicity. Eighteen pharmaceutical companies in the UK, Switzerland and the USA gave information on 29 compounds for which they terminated development between 1975 and 1986. Lumley concluded, from these data, that it was not possible to draw any ocnclusions as to why some adverse reactions were predicted and others were not. More information would be needed–for example, on number of animals, species used, duration of exposure to drug in animals and man, comparative metabolism and pharmacokinetic data, and dose levels in animals and man. Without these data the predictive value of animal studies for man was doubtful.

Heywood (1990) has commented that many adverse reactions in man–in particular, immunotoxicity, allergy, hypersensitivity and effects on bone marrow–are unpredictable in animal models. The correlation between target system toxicity in the rat and a non-rodent species is around 30 per cent and the best guess for the correlation of adverse reactions in man and animal toxicity data is somewhere between 5 and 25 per cent.

Harmonization of Regulations–Reduced Number

The International Conference on Harmonization of Technial Requirements for Registration of Pharmaceuticals for Human Use, held in Brussels from 5 to 7 November 1991, has had important implications for animal safety testing. This tripartite conference, representing mainly the Commission of the European Communities, the US Food and Drug Administration and the Japanese Ministry of Health and Welfare, together with the pharmaceutical industry as represented by the International Federation of Pharmaceutical Manufacturers Associations, the European Federation of Pharmaceutical Industry Associations, the US Pharmaceutical Manufacturers Association and the Japanese Pharmaceutical Manufacturers Association, discussed harmonization of regulatory requirements between the three regions the USA, the European Community and Japan. The Conference was preceded by 2 years of preaparatory technical discussions aimed at ensuring that good-quality, safe and effective medicines are developed and registered in the most efficient and cost-effective manner. Within this objective there was an intent to minimize the use of animal testing without compromising the regulatory obligations of safety and effectiveness. These recommendations should be adopted within a short period, with considerable savings in resources and the number of animals used.

In the Workshop on Safety, agreement was reached on all aspects of single-dose studies–in particular, on dropping LD_{50} determination. The tests which will replace the determination of LD_{50} will have a testing protocol which uses the fewest number of animals possible for the approximation of the highest non-lethal or the lowest lethal dose. In the area of repeated-dose safety studies, agreement was reached on the questions of delayed toxicity and appropriate dosing levels as well as on the reduction from 12 to 6 months duration for long-term studies. In specific circumstances, in non-rodents, 12 month studies may be requested.

In the area of reproductive toxicity, the existing guidelines were regarded as equivalent and, in addition, a tripartite guideline will be recommended in 1992.

For safety studies in biotechnology is emerged from the scientific discussions that requirements are equivalent and the major points of convergence were underlined.

Discussions on timing of toxicity studies versus clinical trials, and appropriate exposures for carcingencity studies, were productive, and harmonized regulations will be made within 2 years.

The Numbers Game

With all the reports on ADRs that appear in the literature each year from official drug regulatory bodies and from investigating clinicians, it may be difficult to understand why toxic reactions to drugs are so often undetected initially. Some individual reasons for this can be pinpointed: for example, in most clinical trials on new drugs patients are usually selected by criteria which may differ from those of patients treated in later clinical practice. Drugs which are to be mainly used in the very old are commonly tested on much younger populations (e.g.

benoxaprofen) and drugs considered safe or effective in younger adults may be neither in the very old.

The 'numbers game, probably exerts influence as well. If an ADR is likely to occur in x per cent of patients, then there is no guarantee that this probability will be uniformly distributed among the finite and relatively small population that is involved in the typical clinical trial. It is only when a larger population of patients are involved that the true extent o the x percentage is revealed.

Do Medicines Regulations Protect The Public But Hinder Research?

Grifin (1989) holds that medicines regulations have safeguarded the public. There is no doubt that the pharmaceutical industry has improved its standards of toxicological screening, clinical pharmacology, pharmacokinetic studies and clinical trial evaluation as a result of the guidelines that have been laid down by the UK regulatory authorities and the Committee for Properetary Medicinal Products, which was set up in 1975 (Directive 75/319/EEC) and plays an important role in the application of harmonized regulations regarding medicinal products within the EEC. It is Griffin]s personal view that the safety and efficacy of medicinal products have been improved more by the pharmaceutical industry striving to adhere to the standards laid down by the test procedures than as a result of any regulatory scrutiny of the data derived therefrom. He qualifies his view, however, by adding that the fact that data are scrutinized must encourage the adherence to the standards set. He also holds that collection of adverse reaction data is of no value if they are not analysed and interpreted adequately and are then communicated in such a form that they can modify the behaviour of the prescribing doctor.

There has, however, been a price to pay, and it is evident, for example, from a review of licensing applications in the UK during the 1970s that regulation did hinder research. Deregulation, in the form of the Clinical Trial

Exemption scheme, has provided a stimulus to innovation without presenting a hazard to the population. Not only is regulation a deterrent to innovation, but also regulatory delay erodes effective patent term and reduces financial returns. Research initiatives are also reduced by high licensing fees. Futhermore, the existence in Europe of 12 regulatory autorities consumes scarce technical and scientific resources that could be better employed (Griffin, 1991).

How Safe Have New Drugs Been?

Perhaps the final question to be asked in this review is: How safe have drugs been? In this respect, it is worth remembering the words of Inman: 'No worthwhile drug is entirely without risk, but few have been responsible for large-scale disaster's (Inman, 1980). Of the more than 350 new chemical entifies introduced in the United States from 1960 to 1982, only eight were removed from the market for safety reasons. That 22 year record argues that the balance between relative risk and providing new therapies is an excellent one (Spilker and Cuatreacasas, 1990). The predominant objective of all national and international drug regulations is to ensure freedom from undue toxicity (i.e., to ensure the safety) of marketed medicinal products during normal conditions of use. Total safety is probably an untenable goal since the use of any therapeutic agent is invitably attended by a small risk that the patient may react adversely to it. Absolute safety in drug treatment is probably not achieveable, although much can be done, and is being done, to reduce hazard.

4

Toxicological Evaluation of Recombinant DNA

These large-sized molecules can more readily biosynthesized by cellular systems using prokaryotic and eukaryotic cells than by conventional synthetic organic chemistry. Through biotechnology or recobinant DNA-derived proteins, there is the potential to biosynthezine therapeutically molecules both for human and veterinary medicine. The definition of biotechnology is somewhat vague or generic, depending on the bioscientic discipline. However, the NIH Recombinant DNA Advisory Committee (RAC) has defined r-DNA as 'either molecules which are constructed outside living cells by joining natural or synthetic DNA segments of DNA molecules that can replicate in a living cell or DNA molecules that result from their replication.'. Actually, both mammalian and plant cells can be genetically manipulated leading to product that can potentially be very beneficial to society. Such generically engineered molecules must nor only be proven useful or efficacious, but more importantly must be free from overt or serious toxicity.

Biotechnology is not a recent innovation, but it has increased in its degree of biochemical sophistication. There are numerous milestones in biotechnology and genetically engineered products.

The art (or science) of brewing dates back to 7000 BC and is represented by a simple biological system (i.e. yeast) that can convert sugar to ethyl alcohol. In a contemporary sense, present day genetic engineering could not have been possible without the discovery of the double helical nature of DNA by Watson and Crick. The field was further enhanced by the 1973 discovery of prokaryotic restrictions enzyme. Restriction enzymes are rather specific chemical scissors which can be use to cut segments of the DNA molecules. Such segments can subsequently be re-spliced into plasmids that are capable of replicating new or foreign proteins. The discovery of hybridoma technologies led to the production of monoclopnal antibodies which then allowed for a method of detection of genetically engineered molecules.

Recombinant DNA human insulin was the first biopharmaceutical to be approved by the US Food and Drug Administrations (FDA) for the treatment of diabetes mellitus. From a toxicological standpoint this first genetically engineered agent (i.e. hormone) did not pose significant safety issues. In generals, its efficacy and safety (i.e., toxicological testing) was reasonably established despite potential species differences. Another early addition to a genetically engineered hormone was human growth hormone (HGH). While the introduction of genetically engineered drugs was heralded by hormones, subsequent chimeric proteins have begun to involve therapies that extend beyond simple hormone replacements.

Despite a decade of advances in biotechnology, only 12 drugs have been approved for therapeutic use. Nevertheless, more than 100 genetically engineered drugs or vaccines are either in clinical trials or under regulatory review. All of these agents have been subjected to efficacy testing, but more importantly safety or toxicological batteries of preclinical assessments. Such assessments involve both immunological and non-immunological assessment.

Regulatory Considerations

In the USA, the Food and Drug Administration (FDA)

has the regulatory responsibility for approving genetically engineered products, particularly those that are to be used as either diagnostic or therapeutic agents. Approximately 300 monoclonal antibody-based diagnostic kits, about 15 rDNA probes for infectious disease and 12 therapeutic drugs have been approved by the FDA. The US Department of Agriculture (USDA) and the US Environmental Protection Agency (EPA) are other regulatory agencies that become involved of the product is contained in a foodstuff or otherwise might pose an environmental concern. The Bureau of Biological of the FDA is generally responsible for approval of genetically engineered products. By definition, a biological products is 'any virus, therapeutic serum, toxin, antitoxin vaccine , blood, blood component or derivative, allergenic product, or analogous product....applicable to the prevention, treatment or cure of diseases or injuries of man'. The FDA applies the same regulations and standards for a IND (Investigational New Drug) for a biological as it does for a drug. Likewise good manufacturing practices (GMP's) apply to though biological and drugs (Miller and Young 1988).

The approval of rDNA-derived products sometimes represents some unique criteria. It is possible that the recombinant's product may differ in molecular structure from that of the natural substances. Thus, certain human recombinant growth hormones contain an extra N-terminal amino acid (e.g. methoionine). Conversely, bacterial-produced recombinant products may have the same amino acid sequence as the natural product, but the molecular stoichiometry might differ. It is not uncommon for large protein-like molecules to fold or otherwise assume non-physiological conformational orientations. It is also possible for genetic variants of recombinant proteins to occur during fermentation, processes leading to mutations in the gene's coding sequences. Similarly, fermentation processes may produce partial products or peptides that can potentially evoke toxicological responses. Documentation of biosynthetic agents through rDNA technology should fulfill requirements for documentation for new drugs produced by more conventional methodologies (Sjodin, 1988). The identity, purity and reproducible quality of the recombinant product must be established and documented. Toxicological or safety testing must be appropriately applied to batches of product.

Toxicity testing on recombinant products includes the customary clinical chemistry and histopathology. A sensitive and quantitative analysis of circulating antibodies is required. In fact, a highly specific monoclonal antibody (Mab) must be developed very early in order to monitor the biodistribution of the recombinant product, both for pharmacokinetic and toxicokinetic information. Test for immunotoxicity is important for FDA submissions for recombinant products. Whether the intended therapeutic use of the recombinant protein product involves a single administration or a multiple administration can affect the agent's potential for immunogenicity.

The phases of drug development for a new drug and for a biological product do not differ to any great extent. These phases consist of the preclinical phase, a clinical investigation of IND phase, the marketing application and the postmarketing phase. The marketing application specified by US Federal Food, Drug and Cosmetic Act is the New Drug Application (NDA). For the biological product or recombinant, the licence application includes both the US Product License Application (PLA) and the Establishment License Application (ELA). Whether a drug or a biological, the issues remain safety, purity, potency and efficacy. There is a harmacological basis for the safety assessment of recombinant human proteins (Cossum, 1989).

General Pharmacological Principles

As the majority of recombinant substances are relatively large protein molecules, there are a number of physicochemical characteristics that must be considered in their pharmacological and toxicological evaluation. Generally, large molecular weight substances are very poorly absorbed by the oral route of administration. For example, either recombinant human insulin or recombinant human growth hormone (HGH) must be administered by a parenteral route of administration thus bypassing the proteolytic environment of the stomach. Because these recombinant products are usually proteins, glycoproteins or peptides, they are often antigenic and hence can provoke immune responses. Finally, blood aminopeptidases and other proteolytic enzymes often result in recombinant proteins having a rather brief biological half-life.

An early consideration in planning for the toxicological assessment of a prospective recombinant substance is the therapeutic use of the product. Diagnostic recombinant products (e.g., monoclonal antibody kits) are non-invasive and requires less rigorous toxicological evaluation. Replacement products (i.e. hormones), such as insulin or HGH, represent physiological supplements and hence reduce the likelihood of suprapharmacological levels causing side-effects. Also, the replacement of otherwise physiologically active substances minimizes provocation of the immune system. Substances that require multiple injections to achieve a desired therapeutic effect (e.g. immunomodulators), particularly if they do not mimic a physiological mediator, are prone to alter the immune system.

Pretest considerations for assessing the toxicology of recombinant sustenance include factors ranging from physicochemical properties to selecting the most suitable animal model. During the early discovery or advent of recombinant technologies, it was often difficult to secure sufficient amounts of the potential product and hence it was necessary to resort to *in vitro* test systems or small animals. Increasingly, gene implications systems have been incorporated into the replication clones so that reasonably sufficient amounts of end-product are now available. With newer recombinant products, it has also not always been possible to identifying a comparable prototype.

Some recombinant products have vastly different pharmacological profiles. While they may all be represented as protein substances, they have different onsets of action.

The biological response may be very rapid (e.g., tPA) or it may require years (e.g. HGH before it is pharmacological efficacy is established. Some endpoints used for either pharmacological or toxicological endpoints may be very objective (e.g. blood clotting), while still others may be less objective or even subjective (e.g. immunocodulators). Immunopharmacological agents or agents affecting the immune system may involve many complex biochemical interactions with lymphokines, cytokines, complements, kinins, autacoids and even neripeptides (Pope, 1989).

Toxicological Testing: Cloned Proteins

Proteins that are coincidentally use as drugs (or more appropriately hormones) have been used for many years. Animal-derived proteins (e.g. insulin-ovine, bovine and porcine) have been used therapeutically for several diseases in the medical management of diabetes mellitus. Usually, patients receiving animal insulin possess titres of antibody, but these are seldom either of immunological significance or associated with refractiveness to the hormone. Humans proteins as drugs represent somewhat of a dilemma, in that these same substances become foreign proteins in the experimental animal. Thus species selection takes on an even greater significance in an effort to extrapolate to humans (Marafino *et al.,* 1988). The toxicological testing protocol of a recombinant product should both and immunological evaluation, i.e. safety and a non-immunological evaluation, i.e. safety and efficacy. Immunogenicity testing may involve both *in vitro* and *in vivo* systems. The non-immunological evaluation is product-specific and the animal testing strategy is focused on the therapeutic use of the substance. When the studies begin to examine thee protein's biodistribution, it is usually necessary to have some means of measurement or identification. The development of a radiommunoassay or a specific monoclonal antibody is often the only means for the product's detection.

Alternatively, large protein molecules can be iodinated and hence some insight into their biodistribution can be obtained, but usually not into their metabolic fate. Target organ accumulation (or lack of) can be ascertained with iodinated protein, but may lack some degree of specificity.

Many new drug candidates, both recombinant and others are being developed for the sole therapeutic purpose of affecting the immune system (Norbury, 1985). There is little uniform consensus of what constitutes a general battery of immunotoxicological procedures. The multiplicity of cell types that comprise the immune system precludes the use of a single test that evaluates all of the possible immunological changes. All immunological assays should be supplemented with routine clinical chemistries, haematology and histopathology. Potential allergencity, including both immediate and delayed type hypersensitivity, should be included in the toxicological evaluation. A basis immunotoxi-cological profile should include lymphoproliferation, popliteal lymph node enlargement, antibody response and nature killer cells.

All of these assays represent a reasonable immunotoxicological profile. The National Toxicology Program (NTP) (Luster *et al.,* 1986) has proposed a two-tiered approach to determine immunotoxicity. Tier I, or screen, includes immunopathology, humoral-mediated immunity (IgM antibody plaques), cell-mediated immunity (T cell response to mitogens) and non-specific immunity (natural killer cell activity). Tier II is more comprehensive and includes immunopathology (B and T cell response), humoral-mediated immunity (IgG antibody response), cell-mediated immunity (cytotoxic T cell lysis of tumour cells), non-specific immunity (macrophage function) and host resistance challenge modes (tumour cell, bacterial and viral systems).

Safety Evaluation of Specific Recombinant Products

Insulin represented a relatively easy recobinant product to produce, in that the amino acid sequence had already been established and safety and efficacy did not have to be subject to overly rigorous pharmacological or toxicological evaluation. Nevertheless, recombinant insulin underwent a rather extensive battery of physicochemical and toxicological tests. This battery of physicochemical tests assured molecular integrity and purity. As prokaryotic systems are used, and because this necessitates harvesting the insulin from the *E. coli* by bursting its plasma membranes, testing for endotoxins and/or pyrogens is required. I addition to this battery of tests, metabolic clearances rates of recombinant insulin labelled with radioactive jodine (^{125}I) were compared with ^{125}I-labelled percine insulins. Thus, preclinical toxicological evaluation of recombinant insulin proceeded rapidly to clinical trials and eventual approved by the FDA.

Human Growth Hormone (HGH) and Somatropin

Unlike insulin, which was never in short supply for the treatment of diabetes, human growth hormone had to be obtained from the limited cadaver sources of pituitary glands prior to the advent of recombinant HGH. Similar to insulin, the physiological actions of HGHs were known and hence it was perhaps not subjected to overly rigorous toxicological testing. Another factor that accelerated the cloning of both insulin and HGH was that the amino acid sequences had already been established for each hormone. Such information facilitated molecular confirmation and purity testing. However, HGH is a more complex molecule (Chawai *et al.,* 1983) than insulin and has a considerably larger molecular weight. Initial efforts to clone rHGH resulted in an additional terminal amino acid, methionine. Subsequent safety and efficacy testing comparing methionine HGH with HGH failed to reveal any significant biological difference despite the presence of an additional amino acid.

Despite the established safety of human cadaver GH, several safety and efficacy tests were required for regulatory agency approval of rHGH. The human pituitary dwarf responds only to monkey or human growth hormone. However, several animal species of GH will promote growth the hypophysectomized rat. Hence, this rat model has been used extensively in rHGH assessment.

Recombinant bovine somataotropin (rbSt) has been evaluated with respect to its safety and efficacy in lactating dairy cows (Marcek *et al.,* 1989). The advent of rbSt makes it possible for increased milk production. Toxicological assessments revealed this recombinant hormone not to be a teratogen nor to have any side-effects on the neonate. It is not antigenic, and has little effect on blood chemistry and haematology.

Tissue Plasminogen Activator (tPA) and Clotting Factors

tPA is an endogenous tryspin-like serine protease that is used clinically to lyse blood clots. There are both natural an recombinant 'clot busters'. The pharmacology and therapeutic use of this thrombolytic agent has been extensively reviewed (Collen *et al.,* 1989), rtPA is similar to, or identical with, the physiological plasminogen activators in blood, rtPA does not induce an antibody response and it is more fibrin-specific than most or all other known thrombolytic agents (Collen *et al.,* 1989).

Several safety and efficacy tests were recommended for rtPA. Both rodent and non-rodent species are recommended and at dose projections of one, three and ten times that anticipated for clinical trials. Considerable efforts were devoted to establishing relishing reliable and reproducible quantitative clot dissolution models in rabbits and in dogs. The use of ^{125}I-labelled fibrinogen as a means of monitoring clot dissolution aided in establishing the thromblytic properties of rtPA (Cossum, 1989).

Advances in other recombinant products that affect blood clotting have also been approved for clinical use. Blood clotting factor VIII has been cloned, tested for its safety and efficacy, and approved for clinical use. Likewise, factor VIII: C (antihaemophilic factor) has been cloned and expressed. These complex glycoproteins are subjected to the same rigours purity and stability assurances as other recombinant products. They do, however, necessitate special animal models to determine blood clotting efficacy. Special inbred colonies of dogs that exhibit genetically defective blood clotting disorders can be used to study the effectiveness of recobinant factor VIII and factor VII: C. In both instances it is necessary to develop a specific monoclonal antibody (Mab) to measure these factors.

Erythropoietin (EPO)

EPO is a hormone synthesized primarily by the kidney. It regulates the production of red blood cells by the erythroid marrow. Recombinant human erythropoietin (r-HuEPO) has been cloned and expressed in Chinese hamster ovary. r-HuEPO (Epogen) has now been used clinically for 1-2 years and appears to enhance the quality of life anaemic patients (Winearls, 1989; Evans *et al.,* 1990). Perhaps the most significant milepost in the eventual development of r-HuEPO was establishing a specific radioimmunoassay (RIA) for its detection. This RIA for EPO led to its isolation, fractionation and amino acid sequencing. Both a bioassay and eventually a Mab assay were required for it to be properly evaluated for safety and efficacy. Early bioassays for EPO often involved using the stimuli of anoxia in experimental animals (e.g. mice) for quantifying subsequent increase in red blood cells. Mab assays rendered such bioassays obsolete.

Interferons (INF)

The interferons have been examined for their anticancer and anti-infective properties. Animal models e.g. rhesus monkey) used to evaluate antimalarial and antiviral properties of human interferon gamma (HuINFg) and human interferon alpha no. 2 (HuINFa2) have proved quite useful in toxicological testing (Cossum, 1989). The chimpanzee is a better subhuman primate model than either the rhesus or the cynomolgus, but cost and limited availability precludes their widespread use for safety evaluation of rHuINFs. At least two INFs (e.g. roferon-A and Interon A) have been approved for clinical use.

The preclinical testing and development of INFa2a (Roferon-A) involves a thorough and progressive battery of immunological and nonimmunological evaluations (Trown *et al.,* 1986). Both acute and subchronic toxicity tests were completed in several species including subhuman primates. Preclinical tests not only examined different species but various routes of administration were studies local tolerance tests, dose ranging, reproductive assessment, and reversibility of INF-induced changes were recorded. Of four animal models examined, and after 2-13 weeks of INF administration, antibody titres were detected in the cynomolgus monkey, the guineas pig and the rabbit. Other safety and efficacy evaluations for INF included antitumour activity, *in vitro* antiproliferation studies, inhibition of human tumour colony formation, nude mouse studies and pharmacokinetics in African green monkeys using ELISA.

Unlike evaluating recombinant hormones (e.g. insulin, HgH), some information obtained from the preclinical testing of INF was less meaningful.

Certain human proteins are species-restricted but the fact that INFa2a is a protein this antigenic in experimental animals may have compromised toxicological endpoints. Thus the development of neutralizing antibodies of INFa2a in laboratory animals may not only affect its antiviral and antitumor properties. But they might also mask adverse effects produced by the recombinant product.

Lymphokines

There are a large number of lymphokines (Pope, 1989). Many of these natural products have been studied; others such as inteleukin-2 (IL-2), have been cloned. Human IL-2 has undergone preclinical and clinical testing as an anticancer agent (Winkelhake and Gauny *et al.,* 1990). Initial testing of recombinant lymphokines involves various *in vitro* tests using both normal and neoplastic cell systems. Testing for antineoplastic activity involved in both *in vitro* and *in vivo* tumour models. Recently, at least two recombinant cytokines (G-CSF and GM-CSF) have been undergoing regulatory review for possible approval by the FDA for the treatment of bone marrow suppression associated with cancer therapy (Dozier, 1991). These haematopoietic colony-stimulating factors, granulocyte colony stimulating factor (G-CSF) and granulocytm-acrophage colony stimulating factor (GM-CSF), act as chemical messenger between cells to stimulate the proliferation of blood cell precursors in bone marrow. These recombinant products promote full maturing and functionality of circulating blood cells. GM-CSF (e.g. leukine, prokine) is manufactured using yeast cells to express the GM-CSF gene. The Chinese hamster ovary cell and *E. coli* have also been used to express rGM-CSF.

Growth Factors

There may be as many as 30 or more cellular growth factors (van Brunt and Klausner, 1988). Their nomenclature is often confusing, but they are perhaps best known by their initials, EGF (epidermal growth factor), FGF (fibroblast growth factor), PDGF (platelet derived growth factor), TGF (alpha and beta transforming growth factors and IGF (insulin growth factor). A principal therapeutic interest lies in their wound healing properties. Some may stimulate endothelial cell growth (e.g. capillary growth), and growth of bone and connective tissue. Recombinant EGF has undergone clinical trials for healing corneal transplants and non-healing corneal defects. All of these growth factors represent challenges to the toxicologist to insure the safety and efficacy of the recombinant products.

Acknowledgements

The author expresses his sincere appreciatioon to Mrs. Betty L. Patton and Ms. Kaye Nolan for their excellent editorial asistance in the preparation of this chapter.

5

Responses of the Kidney to Toxic Compounds

A toxic insult to the kidney may affect some or all of these functions but, in general, it is markers of excretory function such as blood urea nitrogen, or creatinine, and the presence of glucose, protein or electrolytes in urine which are commonly monitored as indicators of renal dysfunction.

Renal Structure and Function

The kidney can be divided into two major anatomical areas—the cortex and the medulla. The cortex forms the major part of the kidney and receives most of the blood supply and, hence, nutrients. Thus, when a foreign chemical enters the bloodstream, a high percentage will be delivered to the cortex and, hence, have a greater change of altering cortical function than medullary. Some chemicals, however, will be delivered to the medulla and, because of the anatomy of the vasa rectae and loops of Henle, can become trapped by the countercurrent system in this region of the nephron. Thus, a foreign chemical can achieve relatively high concentrations in the medulla although the blood flow in relatively poor.

The functional anatomy of the kidney is based on the nephron structure which has three separate elements, the vasculature, the glomerulus, the tubular component. All nephrons have their major vascular components and glomeruli in the cortex. The proximal convoluted tubules (pars convoluta) are located in the cortex, with the straight portions of the proximal tubules (pars recta) extending into the outer stripe of the outer medulla. Those nephrons whose glomeruli are close to the cortical surface (cortical nephrons)

Each anatomically distinct part of the nephron has a specific function or function, all of which can be perturbed by a nephrotoxic insult. The vascular component serves to deliver oxygen and vascular component serves to deliver oxygen and metabolic substrates to the nephron for maintenance of its function, while certain end products of metabolism and other materials are delivered to the tubule for excretion. The blood supply also enables reabsorbed materials and those synthesized in the kidney to be returned to the systemic circulation.

The glomerulus contains a very specialized capillary network which is relatively porous and acts as a selective filter of components from plasma. On the basis of molecular weight and net charge, certain materials and chemicals will filtered into the tubular lumen, while others will be retained in the circulation. (See Dworkin and Brenner, 1985, and Maunshach *et al.*, 1980, for more detailed information.) The tubular part of the nephron selectively reabsorbs the majority, about 98 per cent, of the salts and water in the filtrate. In a normal healthy kidney there is almost complete reabsorption of filtered glucose and amino acids and selective elimination of end or waste products of metabolism. The proximal tubule is also able to actively secrete certain chemicals into the urine; the excretion of some organic compounds and the elimination of hydrogen and potassium ions occur primarily via this route. (See Gregeer *et al.*, 1981, Moller and Sheikh, 1983, and Weiner, 1985, for more detailed information.)

Depending on the size of a toxic insult, chemicals may produce changes in renal function which are mild and reversible or which are permanent, and if severe enough they will cause death. For example, nephrotoxicity may be expressed as a minor perturbation in tubular reabsoption such as a mild or tansient glucosuria or proteinuria, as a decreased concentration ability (for example, polyuria) or, following a more severe insult, as acute renal failure associated with anuria and elevations in creatinine and blood urea nitrogen.

Susceptibility of the Kidney to Toxic Insult

The two kidneys comprise about 1 put cent of the body weight, but receive about 25 per cent of the cardiac output, and about one-third of the plasma water that reaches the kidney is faltered. Maintenance of renal function requires delivery of large quantities of oxygen and metabolic substrates to the kidney. Thus, the kidney, especially the pars rects of the proximal tubule, is particularly susceptible to agents that produce cellular anoxia—for instance, a decrease in blood pressure or blood volume, as in shock or haemorrhage (Glaumann and Traump, 1975; Venkatchalam *et al.*, 1978). Similarly, dehydration, due to either increased heat output or decreased water intake, or a chemical which causes a decrease in plasma volume (Lock, 1979) can lead to a marked alteration in renal function.

Potentially toxic chemicals present in the bloodstream will be delivered to the kidneys in large quantities, especially to the cortex, which receives about 80 per cent of the total renal blood flow. This, together with the ability of the kidney to concentrate tubular fluid, may enhance the toxic effect on the proximal tubular cells, by generation a high concentration of the chemical in the tubular lumen. In addition, if a chemical which has been filtered at the glomerulus and concentrated within the tubule is then reabsorbed, by a passive or active mechanism, it will pass through the cells of the nephron at relatively high concentrations and potentially lead to intracellular toxicity. Finally, many organic chemicals undergo active transport from the blood into proximal tubular cells and then diffuse into the tubular human. Thus, the proximal tubular cells can be exposed to higher concentrations than those present in plasma. This active transport occurs in all three segments of the proximal tubule, although considerable variation exists from segment to segment depending on the species (Roch-Ramel and Weiner, 1980; Greger *et al.*, 1981; Weiner, 1985).

The renal medulla receives a much lower blood flow and therefore receives relatively less potential toxic chemical via the bloodstream. However, as the chemical passes down the nephron into the medulla the countercurrent mechanisms may lead to a chemical becoming concentrated in this region and the papilla to a concentration many times greater than that in the plasma (Duggin and Mudge, 1976; Mudge, 1982).

Once a chemical has become concentrated in a renal cell, it may act directly or require further metabolism to produce a toxic response. A direct acting chemical presumably acts by interfering with important metabolic events—for instance, inhibition of mitochondrial function of key enzymes involved in energy metabolism. Alternatively, the chemical may be converted to a reactive species that may bind covalently to critical sites in proteins or initiate lipid protestation leading to cellular damage. In the latter case the chemical could have already undergone metabolism in another organ and the stable metabolite have entered the kidney where further metabolism to generate a reactive species occurs.

Most of the common enzymes involved in the metabolism of foreign compounds, such as cytochrome(s) P-450 and glutathions-S-transferases, are present in renal tissue, although the specific activities of these enzymes are usually lower than that found in the live (Anders, 1980). However, the nephron has a very marked cellular heterogeneity and there are major differences in the relative amounts of certain enzymes in the different regions of the nephron (Gurder and Ross, 1984). Thus, any measurement of enzyme activities in whole kidney as opposed to renal cortex or medulla or isolated glomeruli or proximal tubular cells can grossly underestimate the metabolic capabilities of these regions of the kidney. As a foreign chemical passes down the nephron, it may undergo metabolism by number of different enzymes. For example, paracetamol, on entering a proximal tubular cell, may undergo oxidation by cytochromes P-450, whereas once it has entered the medulla, it can undergo co-oxidation via the endoperoxidase synthetase pathway (Mohandas *et at.*, 1981). Frequently the intrarenal location of injury represents the site of accumulation of either the chemical or its metabolite, or the location of the enzymes which are responsible for activating it.

Measurement of the Effect of Chemicals on Renal Function

A number of non-invasive techniques are available to assess whether a chemical has had a marked effect on the kindey in both experimental animals and man. A battery of simple tests has evolved which can be applied to urine to give an indication of renal injury. These measurements can be conducted on a temporal basis during feeding studies in experimental animals, or in man exposed to a potentially harmful compound in the workplace, or during drug therapy. The various advantages and disadvantages of these techniques will not be discussed in detail in this chapter. Readers are referred to the following review articles and papers therein: Stonard, 1987; Dawnay and Cattell, 1987; Lauwerys and Bernary, 1989; Stonard, 1990.

The standard battery of measurements includes urine volume and osmolality, urinary pH and the excretion of the electrolytes Na^{+} and k^{+}. The presence of glucose or excess protein in urine and changes in urinary sediment would all indicate abnormalities in renal function. The increased excretion of specific enzymes of renal origin in urine can indicate abnormality of function. Certain enzymes that increase in the urine can be of postrenal origin—for instance, the bladder—and as such are not indicative of renal damage. However measurement of N-acetyl-b-D-glucosminidase, which is primarily of renal origin, has been successfully used as an early indicator of renal transplant rejection in man (Yuen *et at.*, 1987) and for the detection of chemically induced renal injury in experimental animals as well as man (Price, 1982; Stonard, 1987).

Once an indication of renal dysfunction has been suggested by this simple battery of assays, it may be necessary to examine in more detail this effect on renal function and to quantify this response. More specific information indicating whether the insult has occurred to the proximal tubule and/or the glomerulus can be gained by characterizing the proteins excreted in urine on a molecular weight basis, low-molecular-weight proteinuria being indicative of a tubular site of injury, while excretion of high-molecular-weightprotein (>80.000) is indicative of glomerular injury (Stonard, 1987). High-resolution ^{1}H NMR spectroscopy has also been used to provide an initial biochemical screen for detecting abnormal patterns of metabolites in urine (Bales *et al.*, 1984). Studies in experimental animals have indicated that this technique can provide valuable information regarding the probable site of toxic action of a chemical to the nephron. Proximal tubular toxins produce marked glycosuria, aminoaciduria and lactic aciduria, whereas papillary toxins cause early increases in trimethylamine N-oxide and dimethylamine (Gartland *et al.*, 1989). Small blood samples can be taken at varous times after treatment and the concentration of plasma creatinine or blood urea nitrogen can be monitored to give some indication of altered renal excretory function. Further information of renal function can be obtained by measuring (1) renal clearance of insulin to determine glomerular filtration and (2) renal clearance and excretion of p-aminohippuric acid to determine renal plasma flow, from which renal blood flow can be estimated. Alternatively, radiolabelled microspheres or an electromagnetic flowmeter may be used to specifically measure renal blood flow in experimental animals.

These techniques will enable the detection of abnormal renal function in *vivo*; however, it can be difficult to ascertain whether this malfunction is a direct efect of the chemical or is secondary to altered renal haemodynamics. The toxic effect of chemicals may be evaluated *in vitro* by adding the chemical or its metabolite directly to renal cortical slices or isolated proximal tubular cells/tubules. Alterations in transport of the organic cations tetraethylammonium (TEA) and N-methylnicotinamide (NMN) or the organic anion *p*-aminohippurate (PAH) across the basolateral membrane have been used as indices of nephro-toxicity (Kacew, 1987). Leakage of lactate dehydrogenase, loss of intracellular ATP and altered transport of the non-methabolized sugar α-methyl-glucose have also been used to indicate cytotoxicity.

Histopathological examination of the kidney following exposure can identify structural alterations that may have occurred and will also provide valuable information on the area affected. For instance, light microscopy can identify selective damage to the nephron caused by chromium (pars convoluta), hexachloro-1, 3-butadiene (pars rects) or propyleneimine (papilla). Light microscopy can also provide information concerning the appearance of protein casts, lyosomal involvement, cellular regeneration and repair or the presence of crystals or stones in the kidney or urine. Histochemical and immunocytochmical techniques are also valuable in evaluating the response of the kidney to a toxic insult (Bach et at., 1987). Depending on the objective of the study, electron microscopy can be used to gain information concerning the subcellular localization of the trubular injury or to probe the glomerulus or papilla for changes that may have occurred following exposure to a nephrotoxin. Changes in mitochondria can be easily identified, as can proliferation of smooth endoplasmic reticulum or alterations in the other organelles such as peroxisomes.

Thus, there is a large battery of tests, many non-invasive, some only requiring small blood samples, which can be used to assess alterations in renal function. In experimental animals these findings can be supported by histopathology and *in vitro* studies with renal tissue.

Chemical Induced Renal Injury

This section will discuss certain specific nephrotoxic compounds. These chemicals may act either directly or require metabolism to produce the ultimate nephrotoxin. This metabolism may occur solely in the kidney or may involve initial biotransformation in an extrarenal organ followed by activation in the kidney. In some of these examples alterations in renal function may be secondary to changes in blood pressure or blood volume, or to hormonal or neural effects. It is not the intention of this section to discuss all known chemicals which have been reported to cause renal injury. Instead the focus will be on areas where there is some understanding of the mechanisms of nephrotoxicity.

Heavy Metals

Several heavy metals are nephrotoxic, since the kidney concentrates them prior to excretion and they are potent inhibitors of a lartge number of metabolic processes. However, several mechanisms exist which protect the kidney against heavy metals—for example, the presence of metallo-thionein and other high-affinity metal-binding proteins, and the compartmentalization of the metals into lysosomes. Relatively little is known about the precise biochemical meachanisms of metal transport into proximal renal tubular cells. Specific metal transport systems on the brush border membrane have not been identified. Metals enter proximal tubular cells by endocytosis following the binding of the metal itself of a metalloprotein complex such as Cd-metallo-thionein to the brush border membran (Foulkes, 1988). This endocytotic process is followed by the intracellular release of the metal from the membrane of the protein-metal complex val lysosomal degradation. The distribution of the released metal will then depend on the presence of various high-affinity binding sites or sinks within the cell (Cain, 1987; Fowler *et al.*, 1987; Fowler, 1989).

Low doses of a number of heavy metals produce a similar response–for example, leakage of glucose and amino acids into urine and diuresis. It the dose of metal is increased, then renal tubular necrosis occurs which can lead to renal shutdown, a marked elevation in blood urea and ultimately the death of the animal. The histological pattern of injury is one of necrotic proximal tubules with dilatation of the tubular lumen which contains proteinaceous casts. This necrosis is thought to be due to a combination of ischaemia secondary to vasoconstriction and a direct cytotoxic action of vasoconstriction and a direct cytotoxic action of the heavy metal, since renal ischaemia produced by temporary clamping of the aorta or sustained hypotension causes renal tubular necrosis which is mainly localized to the pars recta region (Glaumann and Trump, 1975; Kreisberg *et al.*, 1976; Ven-katchalam *et al.*, 1978). The fall in blood pressure is thought to trigger the release of renin, which activates angiotensin, a potent vasocon-strictor. The site of renal necrosis produced by ischaemia is the same as that seen with several heavy matals, which suggests a vascular component in the acute renal failure. However, chronic salt loading of rats, which depletes intrarenal renin prior to administration of a heavy metal, can protect against the functional impairment without affecting the extent of necrosis (DiBona *et al.*, 1971; Flamenbaum *et al.*, 1973), which indicates a role for the direct action of heavy metals on the tubular epithelium. There is also frequently a good correlation between the renal localization of a heavy metal and the site of morphological damage. On the basis of the above it seems plausible to conclude that the nephrotoxicity of heavy metals occurs by two distinct mechanisms: (1) acute renal failure mediated through the release of renin, which can be prevented by depletion of intrarenal renin, and (2) proximal tubular necrosis, which seems to be due to accumulation of the metal in the proximal tubular cells.

Inorganic Mercury

Extensive data are available on the nephrotoxicity of

mercuric chloride ($HgCl_2$), primarily because of its use as a model compound to produce acute renal failure in experimental animals. Functional impairment probably results from both vasoconstriction and a direct cytotoxic effect of the metal. Small nephrotoxic doses of $HgCl_2$ produce a selective necrosis histologically located in the pars recta of the proximal tubule (Rhodin and Crowson, 1962; Gritzka and Trump, 1968). The location of the leasion in this region is consistent with the localization of the metal (Taugner *et at.*, 1966). However, as the dose of $HgCl_2$ is increased, the injury extends into the pars convoluta (Rhodin and Crowson, 1962). The basic biochemical mechanism whereby $HgCl_2$ produces renal cellular damage is unclear. $HgCl_2$ will readily react with thiol groups is proteins and enzymes (Webb, 1966) in the latter case, causing inhibition of cellular function. It has, however, been difficult to identify *in vivo* those proteins most sensitive to mercury (Vallee and Ulmer, 1972). The earliest pathological changes following $HgCl_2$ are loss of brush border membranes, dispersion of ribosomes and the clumping of smooth membranes in the cytoplasm (Ganote *et al.*, 1975; McDowell *et al.*, 1976). These changes are followed by the appearance of vacuoles in the cytoplasm and clumping of nuclear chromatin. Rupture of the plasma membrane and mitochondrial changes are late changes associated with the onset of renal necrosis. Histochemical studies have shown that enzyme activities associated with the brush border membrance–e.g. alkaline phosphatase and 5'–nucleotidase– were decreased as early as 15 min following $HgCl_2$ administration (Zalme *et al.*, 1976). Kempson *et al.*, (1977) found a three-fold increase in the urinary excretin of alkaline phosphatase, within 3 h of $HgCl_2$ administration. Thus, the changes following $HgCl_2$ are first associated with the brush border membranes and apical vacuole and only later with mitochondria and other structures within the cell. Procedures for the isolation of brush border membrane vesicles from the kidney have been devised and can be used to study transport of substrates (Boumendil-Podevin and Podevin, 1983). These have been used to examine the effect of a number of heavy metals including $HgCl_2$ on membrane function (Berndt and Ansari, 1990). $HgCl_2$ inhibited glucose transport by brush border vesicles at a time when no effect was seen on basolateral membrane vesicle function, which supports the suggested selective action of metals of membrane fuction.

Organomercurials

The rate of decomposition of organomercurials to form Hg^{2+} appears to reflect the relative nephrotoxicity of these chemicals, the ranking order (from least to most toxic) being $MeHg^+ < EtHg^+ < PhHg^+ < MeoEtHg < Hg^{2+}$ (Magos, 1982). The alkyl mercurials, which decompose quite slowly, can produce renal injury, although their primary action is on the nervous system. For example, the victims of the ethyl mercury epidemics in Iraq showed polyuria or oliguria with urinary casts and excretion of albumin (Jalili and Abbasi, 1961). However, in the large epidemics following methyl mercury exposure the kidneys of even the most severely affected people were spared (Bakir *et al.*, 1973). Nevertheless, chronic administration of methyl mercury will produce renal damage in rats (Fowler, 1972); Magos and Buther, 1972; Klein *et al.*, 1973; Mitsumori *et al.*, 1984) and mice (Mitsumori *et al.*, 1990). Fowler (1972) showed that chronic administration of methyl mercury to rats produced ultrastructural damage to the pars rects of the proximal tubule which included proliferation of smooth endoplasmic reticulum, degeneration of mitochondria and cellular necrosis. These lesions are also seen following inorganic mercury exposure to rats (Rhodin and Crowson, 1962; Gritzka and Trump, 1968), which supports the view that it is the release of inorganic mercury that is responsible for the renal injury. Chronic administration of methyl mercury in the diet for 2 years to mice caused nephropathy and a high incidence of renal tumours in male mice (Mitsumori *et al.*, 1990).

Mercury-induced Glomerulonephritis

Mercury has been reported to produce an

immunologically-mdiated glomerulonephritis in both man and experimental animals (Druet *et al.*, 1987a, b). The cause of this glomerulonephritis is not well understood and different mechanisms may operate depending upon species and strain. Administration of $HgCl_2$ 1 mg kg^{-1} three times a week to the Brown Norway strain of rat produces an autoimmune response with an increase of circulating IgE, IgG and antiglomerular basement membrane antibodies; these latte antibodies can be found deposited along the glomerular capillary wall and this deposition is associated with the occurrence of marked proteinuria and the nephrotic syndrome. This autoimmune disease in the Brown Norway rat is not does-dependent, since lower doses induce the same response, nor does the route of administration (oral, topical or parenteral) influence the response. Also important is the fact that several mercurials ($HgCl_2$, methyl mercury or various pharmaceuticals containing mercury) all induce this response to various degrees. The autoimmune response is under genetic control, the Brown Norway rat being the only strain out of 22 tested which responded. However, glomerular lesions have also been induced with $HgCl_2$ in various other strains of rats, the immune response being different from that seen in the Brown Norway rat. In these strains it was characterized as an immune-complex-type glomerulonephritis with the presence of antinuclear antibodies. It therefore seems that the mechanism responsible for the autoimmune glomerulonephritis can be different, depending on the strain of rat tested. Mercuric chloride will also mice (Roman-Franco *et al.*, 1978; Albini *et al.*, 1982).

Cadmium

Damage to proximal renal tubules is characteristic feature of long-term, but not acute, cadmium exposure in both humans and experimental animals. Acute doses of Cd^{2+} accumulate predominantly in the livery, whereas following chronic exposure in the diet it is the kidney which ultimately accumulates the highest concentration of Cd^{2+}. Cd^{2+} or Cd^{2+} –protein complexes accumulated by hepatic parenchymal cells induce the synthesis of metallo-thionein, a low-molecular-wight cysteine-rich protein, which binds cadmium very avidly. This Cd^{2+}–metallothionein complex is then thought to be very gradually released from the liver and taken up by endocytosis into renal proximal tubular cells, where free Cd^{2+} can be generated due to lysolomal degradation of the complex. The kidney is able to accumulate large concentrations of Cd^{2+} –metallothionein without obvious damage until a critical concentration of between 100 and 200 μg Cd^{2+} g^{-1} renal cortex is attained at which renal injury is initiated (Friberg, 1984). Proximal tubular cells can synthesize metallothionein in response to a rise in intracellular Cd^{2+} concentration and the onset of renal injury may reflect a saturation of all the available binding sites in the cell (both constitutive and induced). The toxic species which precipitates the renal damage is almost certainly free (non-metallothionein-bound) cadmium. It is known that Cd^{2+} *per se* is a very potent inhibitor of enzymes and biochemical pathways, whereas Cd^{2+} –metallothionein is not.

Administration of Cd-metallothionein to rats produces a very marked nephrotoxicity at much lower doses than does Cd^{2+} itself. In this acute model considerably more Cd^{2+} is delivered to the kidney than in the low-level chronic situation such that the defence mechanism(s), e.g. metallothionein, may not be adequately induced to afford protection; Cain (1987) and references therein.

Other Metals

Two other metals which are nephrotoxic should be mentioned–chromium and lead. Acute necrosis of the proximal convoluted tubule has been reported in man following exposure to hexavalent chromium (Cr^{6+}) (Franchini *et al.*, 1978; Jao *et al.*, 1983). Various studies have confirmed these findings in ordents. The primary site of action of Cr^{6+} is the convoluted portin of the proximal tubule (Evan and Dail, 1974; Berndt, 1975), which is different from that seen with mercury. These morphological findings are supported by functional studies where, for example, glucose reabsorption, a function of the convoluted part of the proximal tubule, is severely affected, which leads to marked glucosuria (Berndt, 1975). As with the other metals, the earliest morphological change following Cr^{6+} administration is to the broush border membrane (Evan and Dail, 1974; Kirschbaum *et al.*, 1981), although how the metal is transported into renal cells in nit understood.

Lead is probably the most abundant nephrotoxic metal and because of industrial exposure there are considerable clinical data. Lead-induced nephrotoxicity is characterized morphologically by the presence of lead intranuclear inclusion bodies, karyomegaly, cytomegaly and ultrastructural changes in mitochondria, primarily in the pars recta of the proximal tubule. These changes are accompanied in severe case by functional changes in glucose, amino acid and phosphate reabsorption (Goyer, 1982). Chronic exposure of experimental animals to lead salts produces a similar spectrum of renal changes to those seen in man (Goyer and Rhyne, 1973). The majority of lead present in blood is located in the red cell; only the lead bound to proteins or ligands which are filterable at the glomerulus is available for uptake into renal cells. As with the other metals, lead may enter renal tubular cells via endocytosis and then be released, presumably from secondary Iysosomes. In addition, there is some evidence from in *vitro* studies that lead can enter renal cells by passive diffusion (Vander *et al.*, 1979). Once inside the cell, any free metal with initially bind to certain high-affinity lead-binding proteins which are resent in the kidney in high concentrations. These proteins are thought to carry lead into the nucleus, where *de nove* synthesis of a unique acidic protein results in metal precipitation to form the classical lead intranuclear inclusion bodies.

Entry of lead into the nucleus raises the issue of carcinogenesis. Lifetime exposure to high doses in rats and mice produces an increased incidence of renal adenoma and adenocarcinoma (Choie and Richter, 1980). However, no renal tumours were induced in hamsters or rabbits and the renal tumour incidence in man occupationally exposed to lead is not increased (Goyer, 1982). Mitochondria are extremely sensitive to lead and, following chronic *in vivo* administration, mitochondrial swelling, which is associated with decreased respiratory control, has been reported (Goyer and Krall, 1969; Fowler *et al.*, 1980). Certain enzymes involved in haem biosynthesis are also very sensitive to lead—in particular, δ-aminoaevulimin acid dehydratase. Inhibition of this enzyme *in vivo* results in urinary excretion of δ-aminolaevulinic acid dehydratase. Inhibition of this enzyme *in vivo* results in urinary excretion of δ-aminolaevulinic acid and forms the basis of biological monitoring for lead.

Antineoplastic Agents: Cisplatin

The platinum antitumour drugs—for example, cisplatin (*cis*-dichlorodiammine platinue II)–are widely used for the treatment of a range of cancers (Loethrer and Einhorn, 1984; Rosenberg, 1985) but nephrotoxicity is frequently a side-effect which limits the dosage (Borch, 1987). Clinical manifestation of renal functional impairment includes elevation in blood urea and creatinine, some proteinuria and enzymuria and, in severe cases, the presence of cells and casts in the urine. Electrolyte disturbances are also common, particularly hypomagnesamia, which may be related to impaired renal tubular absorption (Goldstein and Mayor, 1983; Litterst and Weiss, 1987). Histopathology of the human kidney showed focal tubular necrosis primarily to the distal tubule and collecting ducts, with some dilatation of the convoluted tubules and the presence of casts (Gonzalez-Vitale *et al.*, 1977; Dentino *et al.*, 1978). In experimental animals cisplatin produces marked impairment of renal function (Goldstein *et al.*, 1981; Safirstein *et al.*, 1981); however, the onset of this renal lesion is delayed. Following a single dose to the rat, histopathological alterations were minimal over the first 2 days but by day 3 changes to brush border membranes occurred selectively in the pars recta of the proximal tubule. By day 5 the predominant pattern of injury was widespread necrosis to the pars recta of the proximal tubule, which by day 7 had started to show extensive regeneration (Dobyan *et al.*, 1980). No histopathological changes were seen in the distal tubule, in contrast to the findings in man.

The mechanisms underlying cisplatin nephrotoxicity and the basis of the delayed onset of toxicity are not fully understood. The platinum moiety *per se* may not be responsible for the nephrotoxicity, as the *trans* isomer of ciplatin is not nephrotoxic (Daley-Yates and McBrien, 1985). Platinum complexes are characterized by their slow rates of ligand substitution in comparison with other metal complexes. When cisplatin is dissolved in water, the more labile chloride ligands are displaced in a stepwise fashion (Figure 11.6) to for aquated complexes. In plasma at a chloride concentration of 110 mM, cisplatin would be expected to exist predominantly as the neutral dichloro complex. In contrast, the aquated species would be expected to dominate at the lower chloride concentration of the cytosol. An important property of the aquated platinum complexes is that the water ligands are far more reactive than the chloride ligands and are readily replaced by a variety of biological nucleophiles. Cisplatin itself as well as the aquated species will readily react with thiol groups in proteins (enzymes) and with glutathione, cysteine and methionine. Thus, a metabolite of cisplatin rather than the platinum moiety itself may mediate the nephrotoxicity of the drug.

Selenium (Baldew *et al.*, 1989) and a number of thiol ligands such as glutathione, diethyldithi-ocarbamate (Borch and Markman, 1989), 4-methylthiobenzoic acid (Boogaard *et al.*, 1991a) and metallothionein (Boogaard *et al.*, 1991b) have been shown to afford some protection against the nephrotoxicity produced by cisplatin. Similarly, administration of cisplatin in hypertonic saline reduced the nephrotoxicity and lowered kidney platinum concentrations in both rat (Litterst, 1981) and man (Borch and Markman, 1989). Thus, the data suggest that the retention of platinum or an aquated platinum complex in renal tubular cells and its reactivity with cellular nucleophiles may account for the nephrotoxicity.

Immunosuppressive Agents: Cyclosporin A

Cyclosporin A is a highly lipophilic, cyclic undecapeptide of fungal origin immunosuppressive activity. It is widely used in renal and bone marrow transplantation. The major clinical problem associated with cyclosporin A usage is nephrotoxicity, which is manifested as a decreases in glomerular filtration rate (GFR). This effect is in part due to altered renal haemodynamics; several studies in experimental animals (Murray *et al.*, 1985; Barros *et al.*, 1987; Whiting and Thomson, 1989) and man (Myers *et al.*, 1984; Curtis *et al.*, 1986) have shown that cyclosporin A causes an increase in renal vascular resistance and a reduction in renal blood flow. Cyclosporin A causes both acute and chronic toxicity, and these may occur by different mechanisms. The mechanisms underlying the altered renal function are unclear but studies have focused on factors that control renal haemodynamics; eicosanoids, the renin-angiotensin system, and the renal sympathetic nervous system (see Whiting and Thomson, 1989, for a review). For example, cycloporin A increases the level of the vasoconstrictor eicosanoid thromboxane A_2 in rat urine (Kawaguchi *et al.*, 1985; Perico *et al.*, 1986) and administration of thromboxane synthetase inhibitors can ameliorate the nephrotoxicity (Smeesters *et al.*, 1988 Grieve *et al.*, 1990). This treatment does not, however, normalize GFR, which suggests that other factors are also involved. Administration of angiotensin converting enzyme inhibitors such as captopril to cyclosporin-treated rats also improved renal function, although evidence for the involvment of angiotensin II in the pathogenesis is not well established. The acute haemodynamic effects of cyclosporin A can also be abolished by the concomitant infusion of phenoxybenzamine or by renal denervation, which suggests that the increase in renal vascular resistance may be mediated in part by circulating catecholamines and/or the renal sympathetic nervous system (Murray *et al.*, 1985).

Morphological studies of experimental acute cyclosporin A nephrotoxicits have show early sublethal cellular changes confined to the pars recta of the proximal tubule. However, whether these degenerative changes are a direct result of the chemical or are secondary to the ischaemia is currently unclear (Myers, 1986; Mihatsch *et al.*, 1989).

In vitro studies in which cyclosporin A has been added to renal cells have indicated that the chemical can have a direct action on cellular systems. Cyclospoin A will prevent the uptake of glucose by LLC-PK_1 cells (Scoble *et al.*, 1979), which suggests that the glycosuria seen *in vivo* (Grieve *et al.*, 1990) could be due to a direct effect of the chemical. Cyclosporin A has recently been shown to inhibit renal cortical synthesis of DNA, RNA and protein (Buss *et al.*, 1989). Changes in mitochondrial morphology and function following cyclosporin A have also been observed; however, conflicting findings have been reported (Backman *et al.*, 1986; Pfaller *et al.*, 1986; Aupetit *et al.*, 1988; Brokenness and Pfeiffer, 1989) and the precise location of the alteration remains unclear. However, recent studies have shown that cyclosporin A is a potent inhibitor of the mitochondrial matrix enzyme peptidyl-prolyl *cis-trans* isomerase and thereby inhibits mitochondrial membrane transport (Griffiths and Halestrap, 1991). Inhibition of renal mitochondrial peptidyl-prolyl *cis-trans* isomerase may be relevant to the mechanism of nephrotoxicity.

Acute cyclosporin A nephrotoxicity is related to the concentration of the circulating drug. Although it is still unclear as to whether the unchanged drug or a metabolite is responsible for the toxicity, most information supports the view that it is the parent compound (see Burke *et al.*, 1989). There is good evidence that alteration of the hepatic metabolism of cyclosporin A in both man and experimental animals can affect the extent of renal functional impairment. For example, inducers (e.g.phenobarbitone, pheno-barbital) or inhibitors (e.g. ketoconzole) of cyclosporin A metabolism will either lower or raise the cyclosporin A circulating blood level and thereby reduce or potentiate the nephrotoxicity (Burke *et al.*, 1989).

Chronic cyclosprin A nephrotoxicity is characterized by an irreversible and potentially progressive nephropathy

(Hall *et al.*, 1985; Mihatsch *et al.*, 1989). The haemodynamic consequences are a persistent renal vascular resistance associated with a marked decline in GFR and renal blood fiow and systemic hypertension. Morphologically the nephropathy is characterized by a diffuse interstitial fibrosis or striped fibrosis with glomerular and arteriolar thrombi (Mihatsch *et al.*, 1989). Thus cyclosporin A produces marked changes in the renal vasculature and has a direct effect on the proximal tubule, which leads to an alteration in those factors regulating vascular tone.

Therapeutic Agents

Nephrotoxicity related to aminoglycosides is still a major limitation in their clinical use. Kahlmeter and Dahlager (1984) reviewed over 10 000 patients in clinical trials with aminoglycosides and found a frequency of nephrotoxicity resulting from gentamicin and tobramycin of about 14 per cent and from netilmicin and amikacin of 9 per cent. Similarly, Hall *et al.* (1983) reviewed cases of hospital-acquired acute renal fuilure and showed that 11 per cent of over 2000 cases were attributable to aminoglycosides.

The aminoglycosides consist of two or more amino sugars which are cationic at physiological pH joined by a glycosidic linkage to a hexose nucleus. The clinically relevant amino-glyconsides are gentamicin, tobramycin, netilmicin, amikacin, streptomycin and neomycin C. These antibiotics are primarly excreted by glomerular filtration. A small amount of the cationic drug binds to anionic phospholipids (primarily phosphoinositides) located on the brush border membrane of the proximal tubule (Feldman *et al.*, 1982) and the bound aminoglycoside then enters the renal tubular cell by endocytosis and is stored in secondary lysosomes. This process leads to the accumulation of the antibiotic in proximal tubular cells (Silverblatt and Kuehn 1979; Vandewalle *et al.*, 1981), where it can persist for days. Some aminoglycoside may be absorbed from the basolateral membrane, but this represents only a minor contributin to the cellular aminoglycoside concentration (Kaloyanides and Pastoriza-Munoz, 1980). Location of the drug in the pars convoluta and pars recta of the proximal tubule is in agreement with the histopa-thological location of necrosis in this region of the cortex. Ultrastructural examination of the renal cortex showed marked hypertrophy of the lysosomes in the proximal tubule and the presence of concentric lamellar material (Myeloid bodies) within these organelles (Kosek *et al.*, 1974; De Broe *et al.*, 1984).

The earliest functional changes are alterations in renal concentration ability, proteinuia and enzymuria and in acid-base balance (see review by Kaloyanides and Pastoriza-Munoz, 1980; Appel, 1982; Kaloyanides, 1984; Davey and Harpur, 1987; Walker and Duggin, 1988). In addition to renal tubular necrosis, functional and ultrastructural changes occur in the glomerulus, where these polycationic antibiotics may alter the anionic charge of the glomerular endothelium (Appel, 1982; Cojocel *et al.*, 1983).

The biochemical events leading to renal tubular necrosis are believed to be initiated by the binding of the cationic aminoglycoside to negatively charged phospholicpid bilayers. This impairs the degradation of phosphatidylinositol by binding to phosphati-dylinositiol-4,5-bisphosphate and preventing its metablolism to the triphosphate (Kaloyanides and Ramsammy, 1989). The binding of the aminoglycosides also alters the activation and redistribution of the protein kinase C complex. Impairment of phosphoinositide metabolism probably results in altered Ca^{2+} membrane transport, which can lead to cellular injury and slow repair to damaged cell membranes, Calcium has been shown to inhibit the binding of gentamicin to renal membranes, and calcium loading can protect against the renal injury produced by this durg (Humes *et al.*, 1984). Administration of an anionic polypeptide such as poly-L-aspartic acid with gentamicin will protect against the nephrotoxicity (Gibert *et al.*, 1989; Ramsammy *et al.*, 1989). It is believed that poly-L-aspartic acid binds gentamicin, thereby displacing it from negatively charged membrane lipids and relieving the inhibition of phospholipid metabolism. Gentamicin inhibits oxidative phosphorylation in renal cortical mitochondria *in vitro* (simmons *et al.*, 1980). This is probably due to altered mitochondrial calcium transport, which can influence mitochondrial respiration. At concentrations which are found in proximal tubular cells gentamicin will also enhance the generation of hydrogen peroxide by isolated mitochondria (Walker and Shah, 1987). With the formation of hydrogen peroxide, other reactive oxygen species such as superoxide anion and hydroxyl radicals can be produced. Hydroxyl radical scavengers and iron chelators (desferrioxamine) have been shown to protect against the acute renal injury produced by gentamincin (Walker and Duggin, 1988), implicating a role for free radicals in aminoglycoside nephrotoxicity.

Thus, the following cascade of events is though to occur. The drug is filtered at the glomerulus and enters the tubular lumen, where it binds to apical cell membrane phosphoinositols. These complexes undergo endocytosis, thereby developing high intracellular concentrations of the antibiotic, and become incorporated into lysosomes and inhibit phospholipid metabolism. Interaction with mitochondria can lead to generation of reactive oxygen species that can alter cellular function and lead to necrosis. The balance between the repair of the cellular injury and the extent and duration of the necurosis determines the extext of the renal failure.

β-Lactam Antibiotics

The β-lactam antibiotics include the penicillins, cephalosporins, carbapenems and several structurally related compounds. With the exception of guanylureido-penicillin, none of the penicillins are directly nephrotoxic. However, at least two cephalosporins (cephaloridine and cephaloglycin) and a carbapenem (imipenem) have proved to be highly nephrotoxic, while several other cephalosporins and cabapenems have mild to moderate nephrotoxicity.

The cephalosporins have two side-group sub-stituents on the β-lactam structure designated R_1 and R_2 (Figure 11.9) those that are nephrotoxic do not share common or even similar R_1 or R_2 groups, although no cephalosporin with R_2 = H is nephrotoxic. One common feature of the nephrotoxic cephalosporins is a comparatively unstable bond between the β-lactam ring and the R_2 substituent which favours release of the R_2 groups. The acylating potential of the leaving groups is an important factor in determining nephrotoxicity (Tune, 1986).

Cephaloridine causes renal tubular injury in both experimental animals and man which is characterized by a decreased GFR, glycosuria, enzymuria and proteinuria. These changes are frequently acoompanied by histological evidence of necrosis to the proximal convoluted tubule (Silverblatt *et al.*, 1970). Cephaloridine accumulates in the renal cortex to a much greater extent than in other organs (Wold, 1981; Turne, 1982) and the extent of this accumulation is species-dependent. Following administration to rabbits, guinea-pigs and rats, the renal cortical cephaloridine concentration was highest in reabbit and lowest in rat. These findings parallel the susceptibility to nephrotoxicity.

Many cephalosporins are substrates for the organic anion transport system that is located on the basolateral membrane of the proximal tubule. competitive inhibition of this system by probenecid protects against the effects of cephalosporins (Tune and Hsu, 1990). Not only transport into a renal cell but also its rate of efflux into the tubular fluid is an important factor in determining the toxicity. With different β-lactams the renal concentration can very by several orders of magnitude and it is the area under the concentration–time curve (AUC) in the tubular cell that is important with regard to toxicity. For example, β-lactams that are rapidly and efficiently transported across the basolateral membrane and then rapidly transported from the cell into the tubular lumen have comparatively low AUCs–e.g. cephalothin and cefaclor. Lower rates of secretion can be caused either by restricted movement from the cell into the tubular lumen giving very high AUCs (e.g. cephaloridine) or by little or no secretory transport into the cell, resulting in very low intracellular antibiotic concentrations (e.g. ceftazidime). As a consequence of these widely different intracellular AUCs, cephaloridine is very toxic and ceftazidime non-toxic to the kidney.

The nephrotoxic β-lactams share two important properties, one or both of which are lacking in the non-toxic β-lactams (Tune, 1986). The first, as discussed above, is the ability to concentrate within cells in the proximal tubule and the second is their acylating potential. For example, the nephrotoxic β-lactam cephaloglycin covalently binds to proteins within renal tubular cells to a far greater extent than do the non-toxic β-lactams such as cephalothin (Browning and Tune, 1983). Consistent with this is the finding that cephaloridine depletes glutathione levels in the renal cortex (Kuo *et al.*, 1983). Prior treatment with agents that deplete glutathione will potentiate the nephrotoxicity of cephaloridine, which suggests that glutathione plays a protective role by scavenging the acylating moiety (Kuo and Hook, 1982). It has been postulated that cephaloridine can generate superoxide anion via a redox cycle, catalysed by NADPH-cytochrome *P*-450 reductase. The superoxide anion formed ultimately leads to lipid peroxidation (Cojocel *et al.*, 1985) and the consequent oxidation of reduced glutathione in the renal cortex. In support of the lipid peroxidation hypothesis are the findigs that animals fed diets defieicent in vitamin E or selenium are more susceptible to the nephrotoxicity of cephaloridine. The lipid peroxidative injury mechanism has been shown to be limited mainly to cephaloridine.

Several lines of study suggest that the toxic cephalosporins and imipenem produce their tubular injury by an action on mitochondria. (1) Respiration is reduced in mitochondria isolated from animals dosed with the nephrotoxic β-lactams. (2) The mitochondrial respiratory toxicity is an early event occurring 0.5–1 h after administration of a single dose; (3) it is associated with a marked depletion of cortical ATP by 1.5 h; and (4) it precedes the first indications of ultrastructural damage by 5 h. The resulting lesion resembles that produced by ischaemic injury to the kidney (Tune, 1986). Recent studies indicate that the nephrotoxic β-lactams selectively acylate and inactivate the transport systems that carry anionic substrates into the mitochondrial matrix.

Paracetamol

Paracetamol (*N*-acetyl-*p*-aminophenol; acetaminopen) is a widely used analgesic and antipyretic drug. It is the major active metabolite of phenacetin, which has been used in analgesic mixtures and implicated in the aetiology of analgesic nephropathy (Duggin, 1980; Bach and Bridges, 1985; Gregg *et al.*, 1989). Large doses of analgesic mixtures containing aspirin and phenacetin given over a prologed period of time produce medullary interstitial nephritis, papillary damage and chronic renal failure in man (Kincaid-smith, 1978).

Paracetamol is capable of producing analgesis nephropathy in rats but only when fed at large doses for long periods of time (Molland, 1978). Paracetamol and its conjugates have been shown to concentrate within cells of the inner medulla rather than plasma or renal cortical cells (Duggin and Mudge, 1976). Dehydration of animals leads to a greater concentration of these chemicals in the medulla, which is consistent with the finding of enhanced toxicity during dehydration. Thus, trapping of paracetamol or its metabolites in the countercurrent concentrating mechanism in the medulla may play a role in the medullary toxicity. The NADPH-independent prostaglandin endoperoxidase synthetase (PES) system containing a fatty acid cyclooxygenase and prostaglandin hydroperoxidase is located predominantly in the inner medulla (Spry *et al.*, 1986). This enzyme complex is able to metabolize paracetamol to generate a reactive metabolite that covalently binds to protein (Boyd and Eling, 1981; Mohandas *et al.*, 1981; Moldeus *et al.*, 1982). Glutathione, antioxidants and inhibitors of PES will reduce the covalent binding of paracetamol to rabbit mediulary tissue (Mohandas *et al.*,

1981; Moldeue *et al.*, 1982). The conversion of paracetamol to its reactive intermediate by PES probably involves a one-electron oxidation and hydrogen abstraction to form the phenoxy radical of paracetamol, which may undergo a further one-electron oxidation ot *N*-acetyl-*p*-benzoquioneimine (NAPQI). NAPQI can either react with glutathione to form a glutathions conjugate or redox cycle and generate oxidized glutathione (Moldeus *et al.*, 1982) (Figure 11.10). This redox cycling could cause a marked depletion of glutathione in the inner renal medulla, since these cells already have a low level of reduced glutathione (Mohandas *et al.*, 1984). The concentration of reduced glutathione is critical in preventing the covalent binding of reactive paracetamol metabolites to renal proteins. When the levels of glutathione are reduced, the reactive metabolite of paracetamol will react with cysteine residues in proteins to form 3-cystein-S-yl-4'-hydroxyaniline adducts (Hoffman *et al.*, 1985). Thus, the available evidence suggests that paracetamol oxicity to the inner renal medulla is probably due to its ability to concentrate in that part of the kidney, and undergo activation via the PES system to NAPQI, which subsequently binds to critical protein thiol groups and ultimately results in cell death.

Compund analgesics containing aspirin and phenacetin have a sysergistic effect on the development of chronic medullary necrosis (Molland, 1978). Aspirin is only a modest inhibitor of the cyclooxygenase component of the PES system; however, it is readily deacetylated to salicylate, which is effective at depleting renal glutathione levels (Duggin, 1980). Thus, the presence of other analgesics may potestiate the medullary toxicity of paracetamol.

In the liver paracetamol undergoes metabolism primarily via conjugation to form the non-toxic glucuronide or sulphate conjugates. However, a small amount undergoes metabolism via cytochrome P-450 to form NAPQI, which can coval-ently bind to critical thiol groups in proteins. Normally this reactive metabolite is conjugated with reduced glutathione to render it non-toxic; however, following large doses of paracetamol the concentration of reduced glutathine in liver cells can be depleted and then toxicits may ensue (Hinson, 1980; Monks and Lau, 1988). Metabolism of paracetamol to a reactive intermediate is also thought to be required for the induction of renal tubular necrosis (McMurtry *et al.*, 1978). Two different mechanisms for the generation of a reactive metabolite within the renal cortex have been proposed. The first is analogous to that reported for the liver, namely that NAPQI is generated via a pathway mediated by cytochrome P-450 mediated in cells in the proximal convoluted tubule. Evidence for this mechanism includes the demonstration of NADPH-dependent covalent binding of paracetamol to renal cortical mirosomes (McMurtry *et al.*, 1978; Mohandas *et al.*, 1981). The second proposed mechanism involves the deacetylation of paracetamol to p-aminophenol. p-aminophenol then undergoes one-electron reduction and hydrogen abstration to form the 4-aminophenoxy radical, which in turn may undergo further oxidation to form p-benzoquinoneimine. Evidence to support this mechanism of activation includes identifi-cation of p-aminophenol an a urinary metabolite of paracetamol (Newton *et al.*, 1982), and the demonstration of NADPH-independent covalent binding of [^{14}C]-ring-labelled but not [^{14}C]-acetyl-labelled paracetamol to renal homogenates (Newton *et al.*, 1983B). p-Aminophenol is about five times more potent as a nephrotoxin than paracetamol, a sigle dose producing a marked renal tubular necrosis.

Thus, there are at least three separate biochemical pathways for the generation of a radical intermediate from paracetamol. The first is mediated by PES, the second by cytochronme *P*-450 and the third by deacetylation.

Halogenated Hydrocarbons

Choroform

Chloroform is both hepatotoxic and nephrotoxic is most mammalian species, including man (Pohl, 1979; Davidson *et al.*, 1982). The magnitude of chloroform-induced nephrotoxicity varies with species, and in mice there are unique six and strain differences, Male ICR mice are susceptible to chloroform-induced renal injury, while female mice are resistant (Smith *et al*.,, 1983, 1984). The renal lesions induced in male mice by acute doses of chloroform include swelling of the tubular epithelium, increased renal weight, marked necrosis of the proximal tubular epithelium and the presence of tubular casts (Hewitt, 1956). Changes in renal function include gluconuria, proteinuria, an elevation of blood urea nitrogen and a decreased secretion of organic anione and cations.

The mechanism of chloroform-induced nephrotoxicity has recently been shown to be similar to that established in the liver–namely generation of phosgene (see Smith, 1986, for a review). Studies with renal cortical slices from rats (Paul and Rubinstein, 1963), and rabbits (Bailie *et al*., 1984) and renal microsomes from male but not female mice (Smith and Hook, 1984) have demonstrated that [^{14}C]-chloroform is metabolized to [^{14}C]O_2, a known degradation product of phosgene. Furthermorc, studies in male mouse renal homogenates showed that phosgene can be trapped by two molecules of glutathione to form diglutathione dithiocarbonate, which undergoes further meta-boilsm to 2-oxothiazolidine-4-carboxylic acid (OTZ) (Branchflower *et al*., 1984; Pohl *et al*., 1984). Administration of chloroform to male mice causes renal glutathione depletion (Branchflower *et al*., 1984), which suggests that phosgene is also formed *in vivio*. Deuterated chloroform is less nephrotoxic than chloroform *in vivio* and in renal slices, which suggests that metabolism is required for toxicity (Ahmadizadeh *et al*., 1981). The metabolism of chloroform requires NADPH and oxygen and can be inhibited by carbon monoxide and metyrapone. Thus, in the kidney chloroform can undergo oxidative dechlorination catalysed by cytochrome *P*-450 (Bailie *et al*., 1984) to given phosgene. This can covalently bind to nucleophiles (glutathione or cellular macromolecules) at or near the site of generation and cause cellular injury.

The marked sex and strain differences in chloroform-induced nephrotoxicity in the mouse (for references see Lock,

1987a) appear to be related to the rate of metabolism via cytochrome *P*-450 (Pohl *et al.*, 1984). The concentration of cytochrome *P*-450 is about fivefold greater in the kidneys of male as compared with female mice (Smith *et al.*, 1984). Castration of male mice converted their pattern of cytochrome *P*-450 expression to that seen in females (Henderson *et al.*, 1990) and reduced their susceptibility to chloroform (Smith *et al.*, 1984). Similarly, testosterone pretreatment of female mice resulted in a suppression of the female cytochrome *P*-450 profile and induction of the male pattern (Henderson *et al.*, 1990), thus rendering them susceptible to the nephrotoxic effects of chloroform (Smith *et al.*, 1984). These findings plus those of Clemens *et al.*, (1979) suggest that the androgen-induced renal susceptibility to chloroform is mediated via the androgen receptor, which may control the expression of cytochrome *P*-450 genes.

In other species the primary target organ for chloroform is the liver, with nephrotoxicity being either absent or only mild. This suggests that perhaps the cytochrome *P*-450 which can metabolize chloroform to phosgene is either absent or present in low concentrations in the kidney of these species. Following chronic low level exposure to chloroform an increased incidence of renal tumours has been reported in male rate and, in one study, in male mice (see Davidson *et al.*, 1982). Whether the mechanism of carcinogenicity is the same as that which produces the acute nephrotoxicity in male mice or is entirely separate is not clear.

Haloalkenes

Hexachloro, 1, 3-butadiene (HCBD) is a by-product formed during the manufacture of chlorinated solvents. The kidney appears to be the primary target for HCBD toxicity in rats, mice and other mammalian species (Lock, 1988). In the rat HCBD produces a well-defined lesion in the pars recta of the proximal tubule, the earliest morphological changes occurring in the mitochondria (Ishmael *et al.*, 1982). The morphological changes are associated with renal functional impairment such as glucosuria, proteinuria and loss of concentrating ability (Lock, 1988).

Treatment with inducers or inhibitors of hepatic and/ or renal cytochrome *P*-450 prior to HCBD administration had little or no effect on the nephrotoxicity (Lock and Ishmael, 1981; Hook *et al.*, 1982). These studies indicated that activation of HCBD by cytochrome *P*-450 was not responsible for the nephrotoxicity. HCBD administration to male rate causes a depletion of hepatic but not renal non-protein sulphydryl content (reduced glutathione). Studies *in vitro* with rat liver microsomes and cytosol indicated that HCBD underwentdirect conjugation with glutathione to form S-(1,2,3,4,4-pentachloro-1,3-butadienyl) glutathione. Administration of PCBD-GSH, or its further metabolites the cysteine conjugate (PCBD-CYS) or mercapturate (PCBD-NAC), or bile from an HCBD-treated rat, all produced necrosis to the pars recta of the proximal tubule, identical with that seen with HCBD (Nash *et al.*, 1984; Ishmael and Lock, 1986). These data suggest that HCBD undergoes conjugation with glutathione in the liver, and is then eliminated in bile. In the bile and gastrointestinal tract it can undergo further metabolism to the PCBD-CYS. Following enterohepatic circulation, it may be delivered unchanged to the kidney or may be N-acetylated in the liver prior to renal uptake. Metabolism of PCBD-GSH may also occur in the brush border of proximal tubular cells to afford PCBD-CYS, prior to renal cell uptake.

The susceptibility of the proximal tubule to glutathione-derived conjugates of HCBD appears to be related to their ability to accumulate in that part of the nephron. PCBD-NAC appears to enter proximal tubular cells via the organic anion transport system (Lock *et at.*, 1986) and treatment of rats with probenecid (an inhibitor of organic anion transport) completely prevents the accumulation and nephrotoxicity of HCBD or PCBD-NAC (Lock and Ishmael, 1985). Once accumulated within the cell, PCBD-NAC undrgoes deacetylation to PCBD-CYS and then becomes covalently bound to renal macromolecules. The engyme responsible for the activation of PCBD-CYS, and indded other haloalkene cysteine conjugates, is cysteine conjugate β-lyase. Metabolism of cysteine conjugates by this enzyme results in the formation of pyruvate, ammonia and an electrophilic mercaptan moiety (see reviews by Anders *et at.*, 1988; Lock, 1988; Dekant *et at.*, 1989, 1990) which will readily react with thiolds (glutathione), intracellular proteins and nucleic acids (Anders *et at.*, 1988; Dekant *et at.*, 1989, 1990). These latter events are believed to account for the cytotoxicity and carcinogenicity of HCBD. The critical proteins with which the reactive moiety interacts have not been identified, but PCBD-CYS impairs mitochondrial function *in vitro* (Jones *et at.*, 1986; Schnellmann *et at.*, 1987a, 1989a), which leads to changes in mitochondrial membrane potential and intracellular calcium levels. Morphological evidence suggests that the mitochondria are early markers of renal damage (Ishmael *et at.*, 1982). The localization of cysteine conjugate β-lyase in the mitochondrion (as well as the cytosol) (Stevens, 1985; Lash *et at.*, 1986) may explain these findings.

Several other halogenated comounds (tri-and perchloroethylene, tetrafluoroethylene, chlorotri-fluoroethylene and dichloroacetylene) have been shown to undergo metabolism via conjugation with glutathione, followed by cysteine conjugate b-lyase mediated activation of the cysteine conjugate to produced renal toxicity (Odum and Green, 1984; Green and Odum, 1985; Dekant *et at.*, 1986, 1989).

Bromobenzene

Bromobenzene is both nephrotoxic and hepatotoxic. The metabolism of bromobenzene is complex, with multiple reactive metabolites being formed, including two epoxides, phenol oxide(s) and quinone and semiquinone forms of both 4-bromocatechol and 2-bromohydroquinone. The hepatotoxicity appears to be due to bromobenzene-3, 4-oxide formation, while the nephrotoxic pathway is via *o*-bromophenol, and 2-bromehydroquinone and its subsequent conjugation with gluatathione (Monks and Lau, 1988). 2-Bromohy-droquinone is a major hepatic microsomal metabolite of both bromobenzene and *o*-bromophenol, and both these metabolites produce renal tubular necrosis in rats (Lau *et at.*, 1984a, b). These results support the hypothesis of Reid (1973) that a nephrotoxic metabolite may be formed in the liver and transported to the kidney. Incubation of either *o*-bromophenol or 2-bromohydroquinone with rat liver microsomes resulted in the formation of several isomeric mono- and disubstituted glutathione conjugates that, when incubated with rat kidney cytosol, resulted in covalent binding (Monks *et at.*, 1985). The role of the glutathione conjugates of 2-bromohydroquinone is further supported by the observation that chemically synthesized 2-bromo-digluathionyl-S-yl) hydroquinone produces proximal tubular necrosis identical with that seen with bromobenzene at a dose which is only 0.3 per cent of that of the parent compound (Monks *et at.*, 1985).

The glutathione conjugates of 2-bromohydro-quinone require further metabolism to their cysteine conjugates to exert their toxicity, since metabolism via γ-glutamyltransferase and the subsequent transport into renal cells is critical to the development of the toxicity (Monks *et at.*, 1988, Monks and Lau, 1990a). However, in contrast to HCBD, metabolism via cysteine conjugate β-lyase does not appear to be involved, as inhibition of this enzyme with aminooxyacetic acid gave only minor protection against 2-bromo hydroqunone nephrotoxicity (Monks *et at.*, 1988). Thus, the mechanism of transport and intracellular bioactivation of 2-bromo-(diglatathionyl-S-yl) hydroquinone appears to be different from that seen with the haloalkene glutathione conjugates. Conversion of the glutathione conjugate of 2-bromohydroquinone to the cysteine conjugate results in the formation of a compound that is more readily oxidized than either 2-bromohydroquinone itself or the gluatathione and mercapturate conjugates. Thus, the nephrotoxicity of 2-bromo-(dicysteinyl-S-yl) hydroquinone appears to lie in its ability to be readily oxidized once inside a renal cell.

The mechanism of cellular injury is unclear, but could be initiated either via covalent binding to critical cellular macromolecules or via the generation of reactive oxygen species during quinone redox cycling. Studies in isolated renal proximal tubular cells with bromohydroquinone have shown that it undergoes activation to a reactive intermediate (2-bromosemiquinone or 2-bromoquinone) that covalently binds to protein, which may results in the observed mitochondrial toxicity and cell death.

Petroleum Hydrocarbons

Acute exposure to unleaded petrol and a variety of light hydrocarbons present in petrol produces a nephropathy in male rats characteized by (1) an excessive accumulation of protein (hyaline droplets) in epithelial cells of the proximal tubule, (2) accumulation of casts at the cortico-medullary junction and (3) evidence of mild tubular regeneration (Swenberg *et al.*, 1989). This nephropathy only occurs in male rats; female rats and mice of either sex to not show any renal pathology. A number of chemicals present in unleaded petrol when tested alone have been shown to produce the nephropathy (Halder *et at.*, 1985) and, in particular, 2,2,4-trimethylpentane and decalin have been used as model compounds. Certain other industrial chemicals (1,4-dichlorobenzene, isophorone), natural products (d-limonene) and pharmaceuticals (levamisole) also produce this male-rat-specific nephropathy. Chronic exposure of male rats to unleaded petrol, 1,4-dichlorobenzene, isophorone or D-limonene ultimately leads to the induction of a low incidence of renal adenomas and carcinomas (swenberg *et at.*, 1989).

Studies on the mechanism of pathogenesis have shown that the protein which accumulates in the proximal tubular cells is α_{2u}-globulin, a low-molecular-weight protein (18 700 daltons) that is synthesized in the liver of adult rats and is freely filtered at the glomerulus (See Swenberg *et at.*, 1989, for references). Female rats excrete less than 1 per cent of the α_{2u}-globulin that male rats excrete (Vandoren *et at.*, 1983). The chemical itself or a metabolite has been shown to bind reversibly to α_{2u}-globulin (Lock *et at.*, 1987; Charbonneau *et at.*, 1989; Lehman-McKeeman *et at.*, 1989) and this chemical–protein complex is then thought to be taken up by the proximal tubular cells (Primarily in the S_2 segment) by endocytosis. These complexes appear to be quite resistant to, or impair, lysosomal degradation, which leads to their accumulation as polyangular droplets. Lysosomal overload is thought to lead to individual cellular necrosis which is follwed by repair and regeneration (Short *et at.*, 1987, 1989). It has been suggested that a sustained increase in renal cell proliferation can promote initiated cells to form preneoplastic foci and lead to renal neoplasia (Swenberg *et at.*, 1989). The development of the renal toxicity and increased cell proliferation is dependent on the presence of α_{2u}-globulin. The NCI Black-Reiter strain of male rat cannot synthesize α_{2u}-globulin and is refractory to the nephroto-xicity (Ridder *et at.*, 1990). Similarly, other species that do not synthesize that protein do not develop the toxicity. Man does not synthesiza α_{2u}-globulin and, by inference, would not be expected to be at risk. However, it is not known whether these hydrocarbons or their metabolites can bind to other low-molecular-weight proteins and, if so, whether the same biochemical events as those observed with α_{2u}-globulin could occur.

Summary

Chemically induced injury to the kidney can occur as a result of the direct effect of a chemical or a metabolte on renal cells in indirectly by altering renal haemodynamics, or by a combination of both. The site along the nephron which is damaged is frequently the site of cellular accumulation of the chemical or a metabolite. Nephrotoxic chemicals may enter renal tubular cells by endocytosis either as the chemical *per se* or a chemical-protein complex. Alternatively, some chemicals are actively transported into renal cells on endogenous transport systems. Once concentrated inside cells, the chemical may be released from its intracellular binding site and cause cytotoxicity. alternatively, renal specific metabolism by enzymes such as cytochrome *P*-450, prosta glandin endoperoxidase synthetase or cysteine conjugate β-lyase may lead to the generation of reactive electophiles that can cause cytotoxicity.

6

Neurotoxicology

Introducation

There are two cell populations in nervous tissue: neurons and glisal cells. Some discussion of their organization is necessary, as neurotoxins have a predilection to injure some cell constituents. Neurons are cells specialized in generation, reception and transfer of information. They interact with other neurons, with muscle cells and with sensory and glandular cells. Information is transmitted by release of neurotransmitter from the presynaptic axeon terminal, the transmitter substance crossing the synaptic cleft and binding to the receptors of the post-synaptic membrane of the following cell.

The neuron has a very characteristic appearance in histological sections, with a perikaryon or soma (Cytoplasm around the nucleus) rich in granular endoplasmic reticulum (Nissl substance) which is the site of protein synthesis. Several short dendrites leave the soma in addition to the axon, which can be very long. The axon has no granular endoplasmic reticulum, and its cytoskeleton has neurofilaments and microtubules which are the rails for bidirectional transport of molecules and cellular organelles. At its synaptic ending, the axon may endocytose neuro-toxins, viruses as well as neurotransmitters, and allow them to enter the nerve cell, to join the perikaryon by retograde transport.

The glial cells include the macroglia (astrocytes and oligodendrocytes) and microglia. The macroglia is of the same embryological origin as the neuron, while the microglia is of mesenchymal origin, as are endothelial cells. The axion is very often in close relation with oligodendroglial cells in the central nervous system (CNS) or with Schwann cells in the peripheral nervous sytem (PNS). These cells are responsible for myelination. Astrocytes are star-shaped cells, the processes of which are often in close relation with endothelial cells and also meningeal cells which cover the central nervous system. A trophic and an axonal guiding role has been attributed to them. It also seems that they transmit chemical factors which give rise to the blood-brain barrier (BBB) in endothelial cells. The mircroglia is a type of resident macrophagocytic cell that can become active as a result of damage.

The Blood-Brain Barrier

This barrier between the blood and the central nervous system plays an essential role in the selection of molecules that enter the nervous system. It is formed by the non-fenestrated endothelial cells of brain microvessels which differ from other endothelial cells in several ways. These non-fen-estrated endothelial cells are bound to other endothelial cells by tight junctions which provent the entry of proteins and other water-soluble substances of low molecular weight. Vesicular transfer, which exists in other endothelial cells, is very low. The endothelial cells of capillaries are sur-rounded by a basal lamina which also encloses pericytes. Formation of the blood-brain barrier (BBB) occurs during development by astrocytic induction (for review, see Risau and Wolburg, 1990).

There are some areas of the CNS without a blood-brain barrier–namely the choroid plexus, neurohypophysis, eminentia media, pineal gland, area postrema and subfornical organ. The capillaries of these areas have a fenestrated endothelium, but there are tight junctions between the ependymal cells.

In brain, fluid compartments, containing CSF,

communicate with the brain extracellular space, the CSF being secreted mainal by the choroid plexus. The CSF fills the ventricles, which are lined with ependymal cells (a variety of macroglia), and the subarachnoid space, which separates the pia mater from the arachnoid. The meningeal barrier is situated in a layer of specialized cells at the border of the arachnoid membrane with the dura mater (Nabeshima *et al.*, 1975).

Sensory and autonomous ganglia are not protected by the BBB, their neurons thus being particularly exposed to neurotoxins. However, the peripheral nerve has a barrier isolating it from the environment: the perineurium forming a connective tissue sheath. The inner layers of perineurial cells are connected by tight junctions (Rechthand and Rapoport, 1987). In addition, a blood-nerve barrier is provided by capillary and endothelial cells which are bound by tight junctions.

Neurotoxins and Cell Permeability

The target of a neurotoxin can be either on the cell surface (the plasma membrane) or inside the cell. As in other tissues, the permeability is proportional to the lipid/water partition confficient, and lipophilic substances are able passively to diffuse through the lipid bilayer, an essential structure of biological membranes. Lipophilic substances which pass via a vascular route can reach the parenchyma of the nervous system and act upon neurons and glial cells.

A lipid abnormality can cause an alteration in the function of membranes and a greater sensitivity to toxic alterations. Since brain, spinal cord and peripheral nerves are the organs with the highest lipid concentration after adipose tissue, it is evident that lipid solubility of toxic molecules play a fundamental role in neurotoxicolgy. However, one protein, P-glycoprotein, which is present at the BBB, is able to eject lipophilic substances from endothelial cells (Cordon-Cardo *et al.*, 1989).

For hydrophilic molecules and effective transmembrane transport can exist only if there are selective carriers or channels (for ions) in the plasma membrane. Hydrophilic toxic molecules can be transported by these carriers to have an action on them, or bind to protein receptor or to ionic channels. The interaction with a receptor can trigger an intracellular response.

Cellular and Molecular Targets for Neurotoxins

A substance is neurotoxic when it causes a pathological modification of the function of the nervous system by interaction with one or more type of constituent cell (neurons, glial cells, endothelial cells). Neurotoxins may have a variety of origins; they may be biological, or inorganic or organic chemicals. In extreme instances neurotoxins can cause cellular death, and when this cellular death involves the neurons, the intoxication can have serious consequences, as there is no renewal of neurons after birth. Finally, neurotoxins can affect the evolution of several types of glial cells: microglial cells which can multiply and clear the organism of debris and astrocytes which can divide and heal damaged regions.

Neurotoxins can be classified according to their targets or according to their functions. Some neurotoxins are active on the CNS regions or on the PNS. Others are ototoxic and/ or vestibulotoxic or oculotoxic. Some act one specific cellular functions. This specificity has been called 'selective cell vulnerability'. Finally, some will act one the developing nervous system. In addition, the type of effect of toxic substances can vary according to the dose.

Neuronal Lesions

The neurotoxins described here will be either those which produce specifically neuronal lesions or those which affect all cells (for example, carbon monoxide) but give a symptomatology which is mainly neuronal, although the histopathological changes can also affect the glial cells. Neurons seem to be very sensitive to neurotoxins, possibly because neuronal dysfunction results in specific signs.

Action on Nucleic Acids

Nearly all deoxyribonucleic acid (DNA) is found in the nucleus, where transcription to messenger ribonucleic acid (mRNA) occurs. mRNA then moves to the cytoplams, where it associates with transfer RNA (tRNA) and ribosomal RNA (rRNA) for protein synthesis. After birth, neurons do not multiply and DNA synthesis stops. One the other hand, glial and endothelial cells continue to divide. Glial cells can occupy considerable areas–for example, after cellular death caused by neurotoxins.

A large number of drugs can interfer with cell division and have been used in cancer treatment. These drugs, in general, are not neurotoxic, as they are excluded from the CNS by the BBB. However, some of them–for example, methotrexate–can show neurotoxicity (due to astrocytic alterations) when administered intrathecally in the treatment of meningeal leukaemia or parenchymal tumours or when administered after irradiation has impaired the BBB. Clinical manifestations are either meningeal irritation, paraparesis or encephalopathy leading in severe cases to coma and death. The neuropathological manifestations are periventricular necrosis, fibrinoid degeneration and small vessed thrombosis. The addition, some drugs that are excluded from the nervous system by the BBB can reach it via unprotected regions, such as sensory ganglia or cells of the circumventricular organs. Doxorubicin (adriamycin) is such a drug, and, while it has not been shown to be harmful in humans, is neurotoxic in animals (Cavanagh, 1986). It induces clear nuclear areas in rat spinal ganglion cells, probably due to a decrease in the size of chromatin areas. There is also a loss of Nissl substance and thus of protein synthesis (Cho *et al.*, 1980). Ciplatin produces similar results.

In the nucleus, actinomycin D can prevent the transcription of DNA into RNA by binding to DNA and inhibiting the action of RNA polymerase. Similarly, amanitine, an alkaloid derived from the toxic mushroom *Amanita phalloides,* inhibits RNA polymerase. These substances cannot cross the BBB *in vion.*

Action of Protein Synthesis

Protein synthesis is carried out in ribosomes, localized to polysomes or in granular endoplasmic reticulum which constitutes the Nissl substance. Methyl mercury acts on protein synthesis and leads to the disappearance of Nissl substance. Autoradiography has shown that methyl mercury inhibits the incorporation of [^{14}C]-leucine into neurons of the CNS. However, the lesions are more extensive in the sensory ganglia which have no BBB.

Action on Energy Metabolism

Sugars and fatty acids are oxidized to H_2O and CO_2 in the mitochondria. Recovery of the available energy is very efficient, but requires the presence of molecular oxygen. The supply of oxygen can be impaired by certain poisons–of example, carbon monoxide. Carbon monoxide binds to metals to form metal carbonyls. It binds reversibly to the iron of haemoglobin, myoglobin and cytochromes, and competes with oxygen on the haemoglobin molecule. It seems that it can also modify the affinity of the remaining sites for their substrate, so that oxygen is delivered to the tissues less easily then under normal conditions.

Carbon monoxide intoxication occurs mainly in attempted surcide and rapidly leads to loss of consciousness. A notable feature is that, when the patient does not die, he or she usually regains consciousness and becomes neurologically normal: but, at a variable time after the intoxication (2-5 weeks), there is often an abrupt deterioration with confusion and cortical dysfunction which may lead to death.

Neuropathological studies show the same modifications as in hypoxic and ischaemic lesions with other causes. When death occurs a few hours after intoxication, there is congestion of brain and meningeal vessels and sometimes small heamorrhages. In patients dying later, there is often brain oedema and lesions of the cortex, and in one half of the cases parenchymal necrosis. There are ofter lesions of the hippocampus and less often of the cerebellum and globus pallidus. Changes in the white matter lesions are also seen with myelinopathy and astrocytosis.

It seems that the toxicity of carbon monoxide depends not only on its competition with oxygen for the binding sites on haemoglobin, but also on an impairment of cerebral perfusion and on oligaemia. These effects have been demonstrated in experimental studies in animals (Ginsberg, 1980).

Energy metabolism can also be modified at the level of enzymes or coenzymes. This can be important for axonal transport which uses proteins (dyneine and kinesine) which require ATP. Some glycolytic enzymes (glyceraldehyde-3-phosphate dehydrogenase, phospho-fructokinase) can be indhibited by neurotoxins. This is true for 2,5- hexanedione (2, 5-HD), carbon disulphide and acrylamide (Spencer *et al.*, 1979), but this process may not be the cause of their neurotoxicity. In addition, some intoxications result in symptoms similar to those of beri-beri, a disease due to a thiamine deficiency (Cavanagh, 1988). Signs and symptoms of this type are seen in arsenic poisoning. Arsenic binds to lipoic acid, which has a role, like thiamine, in pyruvate decarboxylation. Some drugs (nitrofurans and nitroimidazales) also cause a neuropathy which is similar to that observed in thiamine defciency; however, it is not responsive to thiamine therapy. Thallium, which binds to mitochondrial membranes, can also have such an effect. The ATPases are very important enzymes in brains cells, as they are necessary for the formation of action potentials. ATPases have been shown to be inhibited by a rather large number of neurotoxins, but the assays have generally been made *in vitro* and it is difficult to extrapolate to the *in vivo* situation, because the presence of the BBB can greatly modify the concentration of the neurotoxin in *vivo*. Maier and Costa (1990) assayed brain ATPase in animals intoxicated with a single dose of substances known to have an effect on ATPase in *vitro*. They used chlordecone, an organochlorine pesticide, organotins (triethyltin and tributyltin), mercuric chloride and methyl mercury. There was no difference in ATPase activity in treated animals, despite the appearance of neurotoxic symptoms not exhibited by control animals. The metals assayed in brain showed that the concentration was too low to inhibit ATPase. These experiments thus show that although ATPase is easily inhibited *in vitro,* this is not true *in vivo,* at least after only one injection.

Action on the Metabolism of amino Acids

This action occurs mainly through interaction with vitamin B_6 constituents: pyridoxine, pyridoxal, pyridoxamine. When phosphorylated, those substances become important coenzymes in amino acid metabolism. One drug has particularly marked neurotoxicity of this type–nameply isoniazid: (IND; Holtz and Palm, 1964), the hydrazide of isonicotinic acid, a widely used antitiuberculosis drug. INH affects coenzyme synthesis by inhibiting pyridoxal phosphokinase, the enzyme which phosphorylates pyridoxal to pyridoxal phosphate. As INH is a hydrazine, it can also chelate pyridoxal phosphate which can then inhibit pyridoxal phoshokinase more strongly than INH alone. The chelation of pyridoxal phosphate by INH acts on enzyme systems using pyridoxal phosphate as conenzyme, including transamination and decarboxylation. In humans, peripheral neuropathy is th most frequent manifestation of neurotoxicity, and neuropathy is also observed in some experimental studies–for example, in the rat. The neuropathy includes axonal degeneration which is most marked in the distal part of the nerve and is associated with signs of sensory and motor neuropathy. Regeneration rapidly follows degeneration, and the neuropathy can be prevented by the administration of pyridoxine. In humans, convulsions are also sometimes observed with isoniazid. They are probably due to a decreased GABA concentration resulting from inhilbition of glutamate decarboxylase. Convulsions are usually caused by treatment at higher doses than those which cause peripheral neuropathy. It is interesting that excessive ingestion of phyridoxine can also cause a sensory axonal neuropathy.

Action on Synapses

Excitable cells have numerous synaptic contacts. At these junctions neurotransmitters are released and bind to specific receptors. Neurotransmitters are destroyed by enzymatic processes in the synaptic cleft; moreover, transmitters can be inacticvated by endocytosis triggered in the presynaptic membrane. Neurotoxicity can act at the pre- and postsynaptic membrane by the action of false neurotransmitters or of excitatory amino acids. An example of a target for neurotoxins.

Action on the Cytoskeleton and Axonal Transport

The cytoskeleton is a major constituent of the neuronal cytoplasm.There are three types of 'neurofibrils': the microtubules (diameter, 24 nm), the neurofilaments (diameter, 10 nm) and the find (6 nm) actin-like microfilanents.

Intoxication with aluminium results in the abnormal accumulation of neurofilaments in the perinuclear region of neuronal cell processes causing the other cell organelles to be displaced peripherally. In humans it has been shown that dialysis encephalo-pathy, which is a progressive dementia observed in patients undergoing renal dialysis, is probably due to aluminium intoxication, as the plasma and the brain aluminium concentrations in these pathients are considerably increased. Discontinuation of the use of aluminium-containing dialysate has caused a marked decrease in the incidence of this disease. Aluminium has a high affinity for transferrin, an irontransporting protein. It has been suggested that aluminium, bound to this protein, could enter brain by transcytosis, thanks to the presence of an endothelial cell receptor. Morris *et al.*, (1989) showed that the accumulation of aluminium in the brain of a patient with dialysis encephalopath corresponded to the regions of high transferrin receptor density.

Colchicine and Vinca alkaloids (vincristine, vinblastine) produce changes similar to those produced by aluminium, accompanied by the depolymerization of microtubules. Vinca alkaloids and colchicine do not act either on brain or on nerve, which are protected by barriers, but on sensory ganglia Weiss *et al.*, 1974). The toxic action of Vinca alkaloids in other tissues consists of inhibition of the mitotic spindle: hence their utilization as anticancer agents. This activity cannot occur in the nervous system, as neurons do not divide, but these agents dissociate the microtu-bules, an essential element of the axonal cytoskeleton rails allowing anterograde and retrograde transport. Some degree of sensory neuropathy is observed in nearly all patients treated with Vinca alkaloids, and their neurotoxicity limits their therapeutic use. The axon is the highly specialized part of the neuron. It is responsible for generating and propagation bioelectric currents and is also a duct for bidirectional transport.

Proximal Axonopathies

Proximal axonopathies affect the initial segment of the axon where action potentials arise. A toxin that particularly damages this part of the axon is iminodipropionitrile (IDPN), which causes a lesion of slow axonal transport (griffin *et al.*, 1985), with proximal axonal swelling and distal axonal atrophy. This intoxication also induces a proliferation of astrocytic subpial processes and the formation of myelin vacuoles with secondary demyelination.

Distal Axonopathies

Distal axonopathies have been observed in the CNS and in the PNS, and central-peripheral distal axonopathy (Spencer and Schaumbury, 1976) is the name given to a group of toxic metabolic diseases of obscure pathogenesis in which there is symmetrical axional degeneration, beginning distally in long central and peripheral nervous system processes and spreading proximally along these and other shorter processes with time. The reduction in the amount of cytoskeletal transport elements outweighs the modest retardation in transport and results in proximal axonal atrophy.

This was first observed in neuropathies due to organophosphorus compounds. In these neuropathies, organanophophorus compounds phos-phorylate a membrane-bound protein with esterase catalytic activity, the neuropathy target esterase (NTE Johnos, 1990). This protein can be inhibited by two groups of compounds: one is non-neurotoxic and can protect the NTE; the other undergoes a second reaction which has been called aging (Clothier and Johnson, 1980). This modifies the structure of the protein or its environment and leads to neurotoxicity. It has also been shown that the link between distal axonopathies produced by carbon disulphide (CS_2), acrylamide and 2,5-hexanedione (2,5-HD) is the accumulation of 10 nm neurofilaments prior to distal axonal degeneration (Spencer and Schaumburg, 1976). This accumulation of filaments is observed in portions of the axon proximal to nodes of Ranvier and leads to massive axonal swelling. The propensity for change in the distal part of the axon is systemic intoxication can be explained by the toxin inactivating material required for the maintenance of axonal integrity, the neuronal soma being unable to meet the axonal demand for the replacement of this material.

Subacute Myelo-opticoneuropathy

An epidemic of SMON (subacute myelo-opticoneuropathy) occurred in Japan over a long period. Extensive clinical and scientific investigation of this disease showed that it was due to clioquinol, a drug used for the treatment of a wide variety of abdominal disorders. Clioquinol caused abdominal symptoms (different from those it was used to treat) and shortly afterwards neurological symptoms: bilateral ascending parasethesia of the lower extremities and weakness of the lower limbs. There were also increased reflexes in the lower extremities and bladder disturbance while bilateral visual impairment was frequent. Neuropathological studies showed a central distal axonopathy and degenerative changes affecting the visual pathways..

Lesions in Schwann Cells and Oligodendrocytes

Lesions in Schwann cells and oligodendrocytes are very different from those observed in the neuron and mainly affect the myelin sheath. Oligodendrocytes and Schwann cells from a segmented chain of myelin which envelops axons in intimately apposed concentric layers in both the CNS and PNS.

Diphtheria toxin inhibits the synthesis of the proteolipid of myelin and of the basic protein in the Schwann cell. Myelin destruction is not affected. The result is a marked slowing of conduction in affected axons.

Myelin-associated vacuolation is a change induced by many toxic compounds acting on oligodendrocytes. The location of the vacuoles varies, depending on the time-course and severity of the intoxication of the cell. If myelin-associated fluid accumulation reflects effects in the metabolism of oligodendrocytes, then its presence may be taken as a sensitive indicator of oligodendrocyte dysfunction. An example is what is seen in some isoniazid intoxication. We have already seen that isoniazid produces peripheral neuropathy in humans. Experimental animal studies have investigated both peripheral neuropathy (in rats) which can be prevented by pyridoxine, and CNS manifestations (in chicks and dogs) which cannot be prevented by pyridoxine (Blakemore, 1980). Chicks show tremor, ataxia and convulsions. Pathological changes are largely restricted to the white matter of the CNS, the lesions appearing as intense vacuolation which can be seen to be associated with the myelin sheath. Shortly afterwards, myelin sheaths are lost and a marked astrocytosis appears. In the dog the most prominent pathological changes is vacuolation of the white matter, the most common location of these vacuoles being within the myelin sheath arising from the separation of the intraperiod line. Vacuolation also arises from swelling of the cytoplasm of the internal oligodendrocyte tongue, distension of the periaxonal space and focal swelling of the axon.

Changes in oligodendrocytes are most common at high doses. These cells show cytoplamic swelling or nuclear pyknosis which loss of ribosomes, concentration of microtubules and sometimes mitochondrial swelling or the presence of small vacuoles and/or osmiophilic bodies.

Astrocytic hypertrophy is the other prominent change in the CNS of dogs with isoniazid intoxication and either accompanies the white matter vacuolation or is found with a focal distribution in the cortical grey matter. The lesions observed in Cuprizone (biscyclohexanone oxaldihydrazone) intoxication in mice are very similar.

Other substances cause impairment only in the myelin sheath, as, for example, triethyltin (Watanabe, 1980). In the 1950s a veryserious drug intoxication occurred in France due to contamination of diethyltin diiodide (Stalinon) by triethyltin (TET). TET is very neurotoxic: patients had increased intracranial pressure of sudden onset and many died. The neuropathological examination showed severe and widespread oedema in the white matter, Subacute experimental studies with TET in rats showed weakness of the hindlimbs followed by paralysis and later tremor and convulsions. If TET dosing was inter-rupted, the rats recovered and histological examination showed that the predominant change was a diffuse spongiosis of the white matter due to numerous vacuoles. In advanced lesions, histological techniques revealed normally stained myelin forming a spongy array. Neuropathy was also manifested by the separation of the lamellae of the myelin sheaths at the intraperiod line. In TET animals, there was an increase in the water content of the brain and spinal cord associated with an increase in sodium and chloride. Cerebral oedema was not associated with modification of the extracellular space or of the permeability of the BBB to large molecules. Hexachlorophene neurotoxicity is somewhat similar. It has occuasionally been observed in humans mainly after dermal application or after use as an anthelminthic agent. It was observed with greater frequency in premature infants who had been bathed in water which contained hexachlorophene (Towfighi, 1980). In experimental studies, the neuropathological findings in orally dosed animals consist of a diffuse intramyelinic oedema in the CNS and vacuolation of myelin in the PNS of rats of all ages.

Acetyl ethyl tetramethyl tetralin (Spencer *et al.*, 1980)

is used in scent and does not cause toxicity in humans. However, it is neurotoxic in animals, colouring nervouse tissue blue and bringing about vacuolation of myelin. The neuropathology is rather similar to that of TET and hexachlorophene but, in addition to the oedematous vacuoles in the myelin sheath, there is an accumulation of granular inclusions in the neuronal perikarya and in the cytoplasm of glial cells. This poisoning is also characterized by the action of phagocytes of haematological origin on the damaged myelin. Remyelination occurs during the intoxication, which probably means that Schwann cells are not prevented from functioning.

Lesions in Astroctes

There are many toxins that lead to neuronal dysfunction but very few that lead to astrocyte dysfunction. An exception is methionine sulphoximine (MSO), which has been used as an astrocyte toxin. It is an inhibitor of glutamine synthetase, which is immunologically localized only to the astrocytes. The administration of MSO causes an absence of enzyme activity a few hours after administration and afterwards seizures, if the animal is intoxicated with a high dose. Neuro-pathological studies carried out in animals which had not suffered serzures showed development of Alzheimer II-like glia in which astrocytic nuclei were deformed, watery and often surounded by a clear halo. This change was present mainly in the deeper neocortcal layers and was accompanied by an accumulation of glycogen granules which was observed in the superficial layers. Glutamine synthetase is a key enzyme in the glutamate/glutamine pathways, and a possibility raised by Yamamoto *et al.* is that its inhibition leads to an impairment of glutamate metabolism. Glutamate in excess can lead to serzures and this substance is ultimately metabolized via the tricarboxylic cycle, resulting in the accumulation of glycogen; there is also an increase in ammonia.

Another neurotoxin that has an effect on astro-cytes is ouabain, but its neurotoxic effect can only occur after intracerebral injection, as it does not cross the BBB.

Changes in Endothelial Cells

Endothelial cells have a very important role in neurotoxicity because of their tight junctions which amost completely exclude hydrophilic substance that do not have carriers. They can also metabolically alter some lipophilic substances. The endothelium of cerebral microvessels seems to be particularly weak in the thalamus, where microhaemorrhages are frequently observed–for example, in seizures due to convulsants. The other lesions of endothelial cells will be described below.

Example of a Traget for Neurotoxins: The Spinal Cord Motor Neuron

The motor neuron controls muscle function by providing synaptic contact between the axion terminal and striated muscle cells, in the form of the motor endplate or neuromuscular junction. In vertebrates the neurotransmiter is acetylcholine and the synapse is said to be cholinergic. Stimulation of motoneurons causes the liberation of acetlycholine contained in synaptic vesicles by a calcium-dependent process.

Acetylcholine acts on the nicotinic receptor situated on the membrane of the muscle cell. It is destroyed in the synaptic celft by an enzyme, acetlycholinesterase, synthesized in the endoplasmic reticulum of the perikaryon of the neuron.

The different sites of action of neurotoxins in the spinal cord motoneuron are as follows:

* The plasma membrane: tetanus toxin specifically binds to the neuronal surface and is used in immuno-chemistry for distinguishing neurons from non-neuronal cells. Its specific receptor is probably, as with cholera toxin, a ganglioside in the plasma membrane. It modulates the activity of the motoneuron by inhibiting gamma-aminobutyric acid (GABA) and glycine release. This leads to rigidity and muscle spasms.

* The endopasmic reticulum of the perikaryon: organophosphorus compounds and carbamates inhibit acetylcholinesterase activity.
* The axon: a disturbance of transport by IDPN leads to axonal swelling due to neurofilament accumulation in the insertion cone of the axon.
* The level of the nodes of Ranvier, where impulse conduction takes, place; blocking of sodium channels by tetrodotoxin may lead to paralysis.
* The synaptic ending: blocking of the liberation of acetylcholine by botulinum toxin prevents the exocytosis of the transmitter or, the reverse, continuous liberation of acetylcholine by the venonm of the black widow spider.
* The neuromuscular synaptic cleft: lack of breakdown of the liberated acetylcholine due the inhibition of acetylcholinesterase by organosphosphorus compounds leads to fasciculation followed by paralysis.
* The acetylcholine postsynaptic receptors: where the binding by snake venom bungarotoxin leads to paralysis.
* Schwann cells: these form the myelin sheath around the axon, of which the attack by diphtheria toxin causes demyelinization leading to paralysis.

Effect of Neurotoxins On The Blood-Brain Barrier

The BBB is formed by endothelial cells of brain cerebral capillaries which are linked by tight junctions and have a very small vesicular transfer capability. The two plasma membranes of the endothelial cells are not symmetrical and do not have exactly the same carriers. The luminal membrane, on the blood side, has several carriers which are mainly for glucose, ketone bodies and amino acids. There are several carriers for amino acids, one for basic amino acids, one for neutral amino acids transported by the L system, which is sodium-independent, and one for acidic amino acids which are transported by a low-activity system. At the abluminal membrane there are transport systems which are similar to those of the lininal membrane for glucose and for ketone bodies, but they are different for the amino acids. Besides the system for basic amino acids and the L system for neutral amino acids, there are additionally two sodium-dependent systems for neutral amino acids, the A and ASC systems, and a very active sodium-dependent system for glutamic acid. In addition there is Na^+/K^+ ATPase, which creates the sodium gradient.

The BBB can be studied in animal *in vivo* and the unidirectional transfer constant can be determined, but as the BBB is formed by the endothelium of brain microvessels which can be isolated, *in vitro* studies can also be performed: this has the great advantage of giving information on the processes of transport at the abluminal membrane.

The BBB is important in toxicology for the following reasons:

(1) It plays an essential role in preventing a direct passage of substances from blood to brain. Substances in general can enter the brain according to their partition coefficient. Entry is rapid for lipophilic substances, except for those which are excluded by the P-glycoprotein (Cordon Cardo *et al.,* 1989). The degree of entry is very low for hydrophilic substances and for protein bound substances, with The exception of substances bound to proteins which have a receptor on the enothelial cell membrane and thus can enter brain: such a protein in transferrin. Hydrophilic substances can also enter into the few areas without a barrier, such as the circumventricular organs. In these areas there are fenestrated capillaries.

(2) However, thanks to the presence of carriers in its membranes, the BBB allows entry of all the metabolites necessary for brain function. Toxic substances can have an action on these carriers and modify the entry of metabolites into the brain.

(3) Brain endothelial cells contain enzymes which can metabolize some lipophilic toxic substances (Ghersi-

Egea *et al.*, 1988).

(4) Lesions of the endothelial cells can cause impairment of permeability and sometimes brain oedema.

Toxic Alterations to Blood–Brain Transport

These modifications can affect the carriers or the concentration of transported substances.

Mercury

Mercury is a toxic substance which can be in elemental, inorganic or organic form. In can enter the animal or human body via inhalation, by ingestion or through the skin. Mercury vapour is readily oxidized to the mercuric ion in blood or tissue, while with organic mercury cleavage is very low for methyl mercury but higher for ethyl and higher alkyl mercuries. Most patients intoxicated by inorganic mercury are victims of occupational exposure. The critical organ for inorganic mercury is the kidney, but mercury also affects the nervous system, the most characteristic neurological feature being tremor. The nervous system is the principal target of organic mercury, which was responsible for two very serious intoxications. One in Japan, named 'Minamata disease', was caused by eating fish exposed to mercury; the other, in Iraq, was caused by seed grain treated with a methyl mercury fungicide. The main clinical symptoms were sensory and visual disturbance and cerebellar ataxia; tremor was less frequent than in inorganic mercury intoxication. Neuropathology showed cerebral atrophy, predominantly in the occipital lobe, and atrophy of the cerebellar folia with disintegration of granule cells. Among the intoxicated persons were pregnant women. Methyl mercury has been shown to be particularly damaging to the developing nervous system and in this case resulted in encephalopathy in fetuses at doses which did not cause lesions in the mothers.

After a single injection, inorganic mercury is detected in the cerebellar grey matter, the area postrema, the hypothalamus and areas near the ventricles. Organic mercury is believed to enter brain more easily because of its high lipid solubility, but its high uptake may also be due to formation of a complex between mercury and cysteine in blood. This complex may enter the brain by the amino acid carrier for methionine, as the structure of the complex is similar to that of methionine, which is transported by the L system carrier, present in the luminal membrane of the endothelial cell (Aschner and Clarkson, 1988). When methyl mercuy is given orally, its uptake is rather slow. Distribution is relatively uniform, and in dogs predominates in the calcarine cortex and cerebellum. The mercury content in brains of patients with Minamata disease was studied a long time after death in 1979 by electron microscopical X-ray analysis (Shirabe *et al.*, 1979). This showed the mercury to be present in the cytoplasm of the neurons bound the selenium and sulphur.

Methyl mercury has a considerable facility for entering cells and dissolving in membranes. Since both inorganic and organic mercury bind to SH groups it may well be irrelevant for toxicity which form enters the cell provided there is a minimal quantity present. In the damaged CNS the largest neurons tend to survive, seeming to be able to tolerate a much larger amount of mercury than small cells (Cavanagh, 1977). Small neurons have a smaller total number of ribosomes than large neurons and it seems that cell death occurs when a critical proportion of the ribosomes of the cell is damaged by mercury.

Yoshino *et al.* (1966) observed that in animals intoxicated by methyl mercury a plateau in the brain mercury concentration occurred as early as 1 day after the ip injection and before the onset of neurological symptoms, which appeared several days later. For this reason they studied rat brain metabolism both at the neurologically unaffected state and at the affected stage. The only abnormality noticed in the latent stage an inhibition of the incorporation of [U-^{14}C]-leucine into brain cortical proteins. This appeared before the development of neurological signs and symptoms at a time when oxygen consumption, aerobic and anaerobic glycolysis, and sulphydryl enzyme activities were still unchanged.

However, as brain protein synthesis is regulated by amino acid availability, the inhibition of leucine incorporation could be due to a decrease in amino acid blood–brain transport. Steinwall and Olsson (1969) have shown, using a semi-quantitative technique, that blood–brain transport of [^{75}Se]-selenomethionine is decreased in animals receiving mercuric chloride. Pardridge (1976) studied the problem in animals not previously intoxicated, using a quantitative technique with mercury present only in the injection solution. Mercury did not increase the blood–brain transport of sucrose but considerably decreased the transport of cycloleucine and tryptophan. Amino acid transport has also been studied on isolated microvessels (Tayarani *et al.*, 1987). They found that amino acid unptake was normal at mercury doses lower than 10^{-5} M. But at this concentration, similar to that observed in Minamata patients, the uptake of all amino acids was decreased.

Aluminium has also been reported to affect the permeability of the BBB.

Hepatic Encephalopathies

Hepatic encephalopathies have been observed mainly in alcoholic patients, often those with portacaval shunts. These patients have a high level of neutral amino acids in the CSF. Studies of the blood–brain transport of amino acids in rats fitted with a portacaal anastomisis showed a large increase in the transport of neutral L amino acids, while there was a no increase in the transport of basic amino acids (James *et al.,* 1979). It has been suggested that this increase could be due to brain increase in glutamine. The efflux of glutamine from brain could be explained by exchange with the neutral aminot acids.

Enzymes in the Endothelial Cell

The endothelial cells of cerebral microvessels contain a number of enzymes which are not present in other endothelial cells and which can affect neurotoxicity. For example, monoamine oxidase (MAO), known to have a role in monoamine detoxification, has been shown to influence the toxicology of MPTP (1-methyl-4-phenyl-1,2,4,6-tetrahydrophyridine). Parkinsonism usually occurs in old people, but it has been observed in the USA in the very young. They were found to be using a new synthetic heroin contaminated with MPTP (Langston, 1985). Administration of MPTP destroys dopaminergic neurons and causes a Parkinsonain-like syndrome in humans and other primates, but not in rats. It was believed that MPTP neurotoxicity was due to enzymatic oxidation to give 1-methyl-4-phenyldihydrop-yridine ($MPDP^+$), which is further oxidized to MPP^+ (1-methyl-4-phenylpyridinium ion). MPP^+ given systemically is itself not neurotoxic, because it is a polar water-soluble substance and thus unable to cross the BBB. What is surprising is the different susceptibility to MPTP among species. It is not neurotoxic to rats when injected systemically, but is neurotoxic to rats when injected systemically, but is neurotoxic when injected directly in the substantia nigra. Kalaria *et al.* (1987) suspected that the resistance of rats to systemic MPTP could be due to metabolism of MPTP in endothelial cells at the BBB, transforming it into MPP^+. This would prevent it reaching the dopaminergic cells, since it is very hydrophilic, in contrast to MPTP. MAO-B activity was effectively very high in rat cerebral endothelial cells, while it was very low in human cerebral endothelial cells.

The cerebral endothelium contains other enzymes such as acetylcholinesterase, butyrylcholinesterase, gamma-glutamyl transpeptidase or ATPases which may have a role in neurotoxicity, but at the moment they have not been often studied in relation to toxicological problems.

Other enzymes in cerebral microvessels can metabolize lipophilic molecules. NADH, cytochrome *P*-450 reductase, epoxide hydrolase, UDP glycuronosyl transferase, and NADH reductase have been measured by Ghersi-Egea *et al.* (1988). Their inducibility was different from that in liver.

Modification Permeability

The permeability of the BBB can be physiologically modified, by action of adrenergic neurotransmitters (Palmer, 1986). Some drugs, such as antidepressants, have been shown to increase the permeability of the BBB to water, probably by a β-adrenergic mechanism. In addition, the permeability of the BBB can be modified in what is called cerebral vasogenic oedema. Cerebral oedema has been divided into vasogenic oedema, due to an increase in permeability of the BBB, and cytotoxic oedema, due to intra-cellular swelling (Klatzo, 1967). We shall give two examples of vasogenic oedema: convulsions due to organophosphorus compounds and lead intoxication in immature animals.

Modifications Due to Seizures

Convulsive seizures, produced by a large number of epileptogenic agents, can be the cause of BBB lesions. This is the case with cholonesterase inhibitors such as carbamates, including pyridostigmine and physostigmine, which are reversible short-term inhibitors, and the relatively irreversible organophosphorus compounds (OPs) which generally have actions of longer durations. Toxicologically, these substances are important, as they are used in agriculture as insecticides and can also have military applications, as chemical warfare agents. Organsophos-phorus compounds belong to the family of phosphates (paraoxon, parathion, diisopropylphos-phorofluoridate (DFP), tabun) or of methylphosphonates (sarin, soman). The phosphonates are remarkably toxic, causing death after percutaneous administration. Most of them inhibit acetylcholones-terases and non-specific cholinesterases equally but some of them act only on one enzymatic type, those inhibiting the acetylcholinester-ases being the most dangerous. Attempts have been made to localize cholineste-rases using organophoshorus inhibitors labelled with tiritium.

The inhibition of cholinesterases by organophosphorus compounds, leads to a hypercholinergic state, as, when the inhibitor dose is nigh enough, acetylcholine, the transmitter at cholinergic synapses, is no longer hydrolysed. This can result in neuronal death and astrocytic oedema in several cerebral structures but mainly in the hippocampus.

Sezures, with onset at doses near the LD_{50}, are accompanied by a reversible lesion of the BBB. This lesion can be demonstrate in animals by extravasation of a dye, Evans blue, which binds *in vivo* to plasma proteins after iv injection. Leakage of the stained proteins is bilateral and limited to some cerebral areas–for example, the septum and thalamus. It lasts only a few hours and corresponds to cerebral signs of hyperactivity, such as seizures and hyperoxia. OPs cause an astrocytic oedema not only during the convulsive period, but also during the following days, the origin of the oedema being vasogenic. In addition, neuronal death occurs 48–72 h after administration of the toxicant. These neuroanl lesions occur mainly in the hippcampus, where there are no BBB lesions. There is thus no relation between the increase in vascular permeability and the observed neuronal death. The opening of the BBB is therefore due not the inhibition of cholinesterases but to the convulsions. Prior anticonvulsant treatment does not prevent the inhibition of cholinesterases but prevents the opening of the BBB. Recent research shows that populations of non-cholinergic receptors, in particular GABA and dopamine receptors, are modififed by OPs and that for cholinergic receptors the number of muscarinic receptors decreases. Organophosphorus compounds thus have a complex action. The antidote to organophosphorus intoxication is a combination of an anticonvulsant (diazepam), an anticholinergic substance and a reactivator of inhibited acetylcholinesterases.

Modifications in Young Animals

Lead has long been known and utilized by man. It is absorbed by ingestion or inhalation, and transported by blood mainly in the erythrocytes. If lead salts are dissolved in saline and administered by the intra-arterial injection method of Takasato *et al.*, (1984), which avoids mixture with plasma, transport into the CNS is rapid and seems to be effected by passive transport. From plasma, transport is much slower, as lead binds to albumin and cysteine. However, lead transport is much more rapid than that of calcium, with which it dows not seem to interfere. It is possible that transport is linked to the potential difference across the luminal plasma membrane of the endothelium. Lead uptake into brain by this system is reduced by active transport back into the capillary lumen by the Ca^{2+}- ATP-dependent pump (Deane and Bradbury, 1990).

In the nervous system, lead intoxication can give rise to either encephalopathy or peripheral neuropathy. Encepha-lopathy has been rarely observed in adults, and then mostly in those drinking 'moonshine'. But encephalopathy has often been observed in children between 1 and 3 years old, an age when they may eat pigment based paints containing lead. Lead encephalopathy in children generally follows chronic lead poisoning. Typically there is intestinal colic and loos of orientation, followed by stupor, coma and seizures. There is papilloedema, and neurological findings often include blindness. The diagnosis can be made by assay of lead in blood and by the finding of inhibition of aminolaevulinate dehydratase or an accumulation its substrate.

Neuropathology normally shows brain swelling, sometimes with collapsed ventricles. The abnormalities are mainly related to the blood vessels. There is an amorphous acidophilic periodic acid-Schiff (PAS)-positive exudate around blood vessels in the brain, spinal cord and meaninges, and mineralized concretions are visibloe within the vessel wall. In a few cases there are extravasated erythrocytes, while swelling of capillary endothelial cells is often observed and some capillaries are necrotic. These changes are seen throughout the nervous system and in the meninges but are more conspicuous in the cerebrum and the cerebellum. There are foci of astrocytic proliferation, and the white matter and astrocytes appear oedematous, while in some cases there is a variable number of necrotic neurons, especially in the cerebellum. Almost all these ealterations are those of vasogenic cerebral oedema, but there is also slight cytotoxic oedema component. Chelation therapy and supportive measures have reduced mortality from childhood lead encephalopathy to less than 5 per cent. However, morbidity, such as mental retardation, seizures or convulsions, remains high.

A problem that has arisen in the last 15 years is the question of whether elevated lead levels found in a rather high number of children can be responsible for alterations in psychological and classroom performances. This problem was examined by needleman and Gatsonis (1990), who reviewed the studies on the neuropsychological function in many children in which lead was assayed in blood or teeth. They concluded that lead at low doses was associated with a deficit in psychometric intelligence.

Experimental Animal Disease

In all animal studies, the susceptibility to encephalopathy has been found to the higher for young animals than for adult animals. This has been particularly studied in the rate since the description by Pentschew and Garro (1966) of lead encephalography in young rats, who had ingested lead via their mother's milk and developed haemorrhagic encephalopathy mainly in the cerebellum and spinal cord. The encephalpathy was associated with capillary vasculopathy. Dilated capillaries were lined with necrotic endothelial cells and later with a hypertrophic endothelium. There was also brain oediama, which developed after the haemorrhage. This encephalopathy regressed if the young rat did not die during the haemorrhagic period, the brain lesions disappearing in spite of the persistence of a high brain lead level (Lefauconnier *et al.*, 1983).

The characteristics of the BBB change during development and it is possible that lead, for a reason at present unknown, interferes with this development and leads to encephalopathy. Gebhart and Goldstein (1988) have studied bovine adrenal endothelial cells and rat brain astrocytes in culture. They have shown that rat brain astroctyes are more sensitive than endothelial cells to the cytotoxic effect of lead acetate. In coculture the two cell types demonstrated a distinctive cellular organization and the astrocytes were lass sensitive to the cytotoxic effect of lead than when they were cultured alone. The problem is different in lead encephalopathy, but the endothelial cells are perhaps a little further from the astrocytes in young animals than in adults, and when these cells are in closer contact, the pathological changes perhaps decrease.

Effect of Neurotoxins on Membrane Receptors and Carriers

Biological toxins are characterized by great specificity. They interact with various constituents of the neuron and can disturb its various functions, particularly protein synthesis, axonal transport and synaptic transmission. Numerous neurotoxins bind to receptors on the nueronal or the muscular plasma membrane and so can be used as markers for the localization of receptors. They are thus pharmacological agents which allow the molecular approach of the identification of receptors and investigation of their physiology.

Biological neurotoxins originate from vertebrate or invertebrate organisms, from animal venoms, plants, bacteria or fungi. They act in a manner which is now well-known, especially in the case of toxins of animal origin. Many have a spectacular action on the neuromuscular junction and the regional pathology they bring about is particularly well-understood in the case of the motor neuron which innervates muscle fibres.

Bacterial toxins have actions on the plasma membrane of the neuron and in particular on it spresynaptic portion. The two best-known are:

(1) Tetanus toxin from the bacterium *Clostridium tetani* which produces the muscular spasms characteristic of tetanus after contamination of wounds. It binds to

the neuronal plasma membrane; this binding to a specific receptor is used in immunochemistry to identify nerve cells, the receptor being absent on glial cells. After intramuscular injection *in vivo,* the toxin is taken up by the presynaptic endings and is transported by the retrograde axoplasmic flux in the perikaryon of motor neurons. The result of poisoning with tetanus toxin is the loss of control of motor neurons, probably by glycinergic systems.

(2) Botulinum toxin from *Clostridium botulinum,* a species of bacteria which contaminate improperly preserved food. The first signs are cranial nerve pathology, then a bilateral motor deficit and often a respiratory muscle paralysis. Botulinus toxin has a well-known action as an inhibitor of acetylcholine, the transmitter at the neuromuscular junction. Electrophysiological techniques have shown that the toxin blocks the liberation of acetylcholine by making the liberation system less sensitive to excitatory Ca^{2+} ions of the presynaptic transmitter flux. Ricin, from the seeds of castor oil plant, is 100 times less active.

Venom neurotoxins disturb neuromuscular transmission either at the presynaptic level or at the postsynaptic level. Their molecular action is even better known. Some toxins bind to K^+ channels and can be classified into a number of subclasses (Castle *et al.,* 1989). This is the case with apamine (from bee venom), with nojiutoxin (from scorpion venom) and with dendrotoxin (from Momba snake venom). Several toxins extracted from animals or plants bind to the Na^+ channels in the membrane of excitable cells (neurons and muscle cells) and block synaptic transmission. This is the case with saxitoxin and tetrodotoxin. The latter is highly toxic and is found in the organs of fugu (a Japanese fish). This excellent fish is particularly appreciated by the Japanese; it must be prepared by cometent cooks, who remove the organs containing the neurotoxin. Saxitoxin is synthesized by various sea dinoflagellates which can be ingested without any harm by shellfish. These contaiminate shell fish are very toxic for humans. Tetrodotoxin and saxitoxin are very dangerous neurotoxins. It is now known that they prevent the diffusion of Na^+ ions through the transmembrane channels. They constitute valuable tools for molecular biology owing to their selectivity: they allowed the quantification of the sodium channels on excitable cells, the purification of their constitutive protein and the sequencing of the amino acids.

Endogenous and Exogenous Neuroexcitatory Amino Acids

The excitotoxic amino acids are either synthesized in brain (endogenous amino acids) or are transported to brain from the environment (exogenous amino acids). They cause depolarization by acting on excitatory neurotransmitter receptors: NMDA (*N*-methyl-D-aspartic acid), AMPA (5-methyl-4-isoxazole propionic acid), kainatc, L ΛP4 (1-2-amino-4-phosphonobutanoic acid), situated on the soma or the dendrites of the neuron. This depolarization is accompanied by increased membrane permeability of cations, the action of the amino acids ceasing when they are taken up by the membrane. As neurotoxic amino acids act on receptors on the soma or dendrites of the neuron and do not act on the axon, they have been used experimentally as axon-sparing agents.

Endogenous amino acids play a very important role as excitatory neurotransmitters. It has been shown that there is good correspondence between excitatory properties and neurotoxicity because excessive concentrations of an amino acid can cause continuous depolarization and an increase in membrane permeability. This needs energy to restore ionic equilibrium and can also be associated with a large increase in intracellular calcium. Both can be the cause of cellular death (Olney, 1986). Endogenous amino acids can act as neurotoxic substances, because the process of uptake does not work efficiently; in epilepsy a small deficit in the process of uptake can cause an extra cellular accumulation of the amino acids which provoke convulsions. This neurotoxicity has also been shown recently to be a complication of pathologist which are not neurotoxic, such as brain ischeemia, brain hypoxia, and hypoglycaemia. Brain cell degeneration observed in adult onset olivopontocere bellar degeneration (Plaitakis *et al.*, 1982), Huntington's chorea (Beal *et al.*, 1986) and Alzheimer's disease (Maragos *et al.*, 1987) may involve similar processes. These amino acids are:

* L-Glutamic acid, which has been used for a long time as a flavour enhancer; its toxicity was not known. In young animals it causes serious retinal lesions and damage to the arcuate nuclus of the hypothalamus. In adults 'the Chinese restaurant syndrome' seems to be due to monosodium glutamate.
* L-Aspartic acid. This amino acid bound to phynylalanine constitutes aspartame. It has been authorized by regulatory authorities as a sweetner, because of its low toxicity in animal experiments.

Exogenous amino acids can also be neurotoxic in the same way as endogenous amino acids; in fact they can even by more toxic, as they are not taken up by the membranes. The role of the uptake process has been shown, for example, of D-and L-homocysteic acid. The L-amino acid has and uptake process and is much less toxic than the D-amino acid. Whereas endogenous amino acids are synthesized in brain and can thus easily interact with receptors, exogenous amino acids are generally of dietary orgin and are transported in the blood. They must then cross the BBB, which has either a very low carrier-mediated uptake for some acidic amino acids or a very small uptake as a function of their partition coefficient. This is the case for kainic acid, which is an excitotoxic amino acid and causes convulsions when administered systemically. Its blood–brain transport measured *in vivo* is very low, while measurements on isolated microvessels do not show any transport. It is thus an extracellular amino acid. A very toxic amino acid can exert a certain neurotoxicity, even if its partition coefficient is very low. In addition, these amino acids can act on circumventricular organs which have no BBB. Some exogenous amino acids are as follows:

* Kainic acid is a very potent excitotoxic amino acid. It comes from seaweed, which has been used for hundreds of years in the Orient as a home remedy for intestinal worms, but at doses below those causing neurotoxic effects.
* Ibotenic acid is found in some mushrooms and has been used for its fly-killing properties, It is thought to be responsible for the nuerotoxicity of the amanita mushrooms.
* Alanosine is an experimental antibiotic and antileukaemic agent. It is several times more potent than glutamic acid as a neurotoxic agent and slightly less potent than homocysteic acid in immature animals, where it necrotizes neurons in the same regions of brain and retina that are affected by glutamic acid.

Lathyrism is a well-known disease in which there is spastic paraparesis due to pyramidal tract involvement, probably induced by excessive consumption of the vegetable *Lathyrus sativus* in periods of famine. β-*N*-Oxalylamino-L-alanine, an amino acid, has been found to be present in *Lathyrus sativus* and to induce corticospinal dysfunction similar to that seen in animals consuming a fortified diet of this vegetable (spencer *et. al.,* 1986). This amino acid is a potent agonist of the excitatory transmitter glutamate and is probably causally related to lathyrism in man. A disease that occurred in the Chamorro people of the island of Gaum is also possibly due to such a mechanism (transmitter antagonism). After World War II, a disease consisting of, in various degrees, amyotrophic lateral sclerosis, Parkinsonism and dementia, called hereditary paralysis, was frequently observed in these people. During the war they had a high consumption of sago plam seeds (*Cycas cincinalis*) and the frequency of the disease decreased when they changed to American food. Laboratory investigation of the seeds revealed the presence of several substances, including an unusual non-protein amino acid: β-*N*-methylamino-L-alanine. Spencer *et al.,* (1987) studied the effects of this amino acid on monkeys, which developed a disease similar to that observed in man. He speculated that the diseases of the Chamorros were not hereditary, as had been thought, but were elicited by different doses of the cycad toxin. People who had left the island when they were about 20 years old and perefectly healthy to live in the USA, and had not eaten cycad seeds, subsequently developed the disease about 30 years after their arrival in the USA.

Another disease which may occur as a possible consequence of neurotoxicity but not only of a neurotoxic amino acid is Parkinson's disease. This involves abnormally reduced activity of dopaminergic neurons. No cause of this disease is known but it has already been observed in the pathology of the Chamorro people. Moreover, it has also been shown that MPTP could give a symptomatology similar to that of this disease.

An interesting hypothesis has been put forward by Calne *et al.,* (1986): Alzheimer's disease, Parkinson's disease and motor neuron disease are due to environmental damage to specific regions of the CNS which remains subclincial for several decades but makes those affected especially prone to the consequences of age-related neuronal attrition. In support of this hypothesis, Calne *et al.* (1985) reported that four members of a family had been injected with a drug that contained MPTP. Two who had received a high dose had Parkinsonina symptomatology. Two who received a lower dose had absolutely no nuerological sing. They all underwent a PET (positron emission tomography) examination and even the two with no symptomatology had an image every similar to that of Parkinsonism).

'False Neurotranmitters'

It has been shown in animals that certain chemical substances can produce degeneration of either catecholaminergic or serotoninergic neurons, characterized by a transmitter of the monoamine group (catecholaminergic and serotoninergic neuorons). This selective lesioning makes these neurotoxins tools of choice for the production of experimental lesions in these systems.

It is now considered that these substances are 'false neurotransmitters' which enter neurons by the same uptake route as true transmitters, to which they are very similar. As soon as they enter the neuron they are probably degraded into diverse cytotoxic molecules, perhaps by autoxidation with a production of superoxide ion, H_2O_2, or hydroxyl radicals.

The first neurotoxic substance of the monoaminergic system to be discovered was an analogue of dopamine, 6-hydroxydopamne (6-OHDA), which has effects on the sympathetic nervous system (it causes chemical sympathectomy) and on the CNS. This substance also causes denervation of the noradrenaline and dopamine system (Baumgarten *et al.*, 1972).

Two serotoninergic substances have high toxicity: these include 5,6- and 5,7-dihydroxytraptamine (5,6- and 5,7-DHT), which lead to the death of serotoninergic neurons in the CNS by a mechanism probably similar to that of 6-OHDA.

In general, chemical sympathectomy is obtained in laboratory animals after iv injection of a dose of 6-OHDA, which does not seem to have a cytotoxic action on non-catecholaminergic neurons.

However, in the CNS these three neurotoxins behave like dopamine and serotonin and cannot cross the enothelium of cerebral microvessels. In order to produce the lesions, the toxin must be put in direct contact with neurons thought to be catecholaminergic or sertoninergic by intraventricular, intracisternal or intraparenchy-matous administration.

Animal experiments have shown that some substances cause selective neuronal death, allowing identification of neuronal projections. A good example is 3-acetylpyridine (3-AP). It is a highly toxic substance for some cerebral neurons (inferior olive, hypoglossal nucleus). After intraperiotoneal injection 3-AP causes the death of neurons in the inferior olive of the rat. The inferior olive is a structure which innervates the cerebellar cortex (Desclin, 1974) and the climbing fibres degenerate, resulting in a cortex without olivary afferents. This permits analysis of the significance of the climbing fibres in the normal cerebellum.

Conclusion

When the neurotoxic dose is sufficiently high to cause cellular death, a phagocytic process begins. In brain, the destruction is carried out by specialized cells of mesenchymatous origin (microglia). These cells evolve in brain very early in development and remain latent in the cerebral parenchyma. It seems that they are activated by dead elements in their proximity and are perhaps able to change their place in the cerebral parenchyma. They are thus resident cells which become phagocytic.

When neutotoxins cause a lesion in the cerebral microvessels, this is accompanied by micro-haemorrhages, especially in sensory areas such as the thalamus. If the haemorrhage is of sufficient intensity, this may permit circulating monocycles to cross the endothelial barrier, become fixed in the perivascular area and be transformed to active macrophages.

Since we first wrote this chapter it has become rather clear that oxygen radicals play a role in several neurotpathological affections and also in neurotoxicological mechanism. For a review on this subject refer to Lebel and Bondy (1991) and Healliwell (1992).

This review was supported in part by DRET (direction de recherches et etudes techniques grant 91–156.

7

Combustion Toxicology

General Considerations

Combustion toxicology deals with the nature and potential adverse effects of products resulting from the heating or burning of materials, these effects include irritation, incapacitation, toxicity and lethality. Although the major effort has been developed to products generated in accidental fires, adverse effects may also result from exposure to products resulting from heating or burning materials in occupational and domestic situations. Two typical examples of illnesses resulting from the inhalation exposure to products resulting from heating polymers are meat wrappers' 'allergy' and polyfume fever. The former affects some workers wrapping meat in polyvinyl chloride (PVC) film. The source of exposure come from the hot wire cutting (approximately 105 °C) of the film from rolls, heat sealing of the folded film ends, and thermal fixing of an adhesive label to the wrapped product, with the heating element temperature at around 200 °C (Levy, 1988). The major products from hot wire cutting of PVC film include di-2-ethylxyl phthalate and hydrogen chloride, and those from the thermal attachment of labels include dicylohexyl lethalate, phthalic anhydride, cyclohexyl ether and cyclohexyl benzoate (Levy *et al.,* 1978; Vandevort and Brooks, 1979). Affected meat wrappers complain of cough, wheezing, shortness of breath, chest tightness and symptoms and signs from irritation of the eyes and throat. The spectrum of the illness should be interpreted as a complex response to emissions from all phases of the wrapping procedure (Andrasch *et al.,* 1975). Currently it is considered that exposure to the products from beating PVC in meat wrapping environment produces effects compatible with irritation of the eyes and respiratory tract; in those with pre-existing asthma or chronic obstructional airways disease there may be an exacerbation of the condition. The effects produced accord with respiratory tract irritation and hyperactivity; the role of an immunological process (i.e. an asthmatic reaction) is questionable (Brooks, 1983).

Smoke is complex mixture of airborne solid and liquid particulates and gases which are evolved when materials undergo vaporization or thermal decomposition. Thermal decomposition may be conveniently described under the following conditions:

(1) *Anaerobic pyrolysis:* Thermal breakdown and chemical conversion of materials in a low oxygen environment.
(2) *Oxidative pyrolyis:* Thermal breakdown and chemical conversion of materials in a normal oxygen environment in the absence of flaming ('smouldering').
(3) *Flaming combustion :* Thermal breakdown and chemical conversion of materials in a normal oxygen enviornment in the presence of flaming.

All these process may be operating at the same time at different geographical regions in a fire, or one my predominate. Pyrolysis is usually defined as the thermal degradation of a material at a temperature below the autoignition temperature. Flaming is the highly efficient burning of a material above the autoignition temperature in the presence of sufficient oxygen. Thermolysis is a generic term covering flaming, pyrolysis and smouldering.

The atmosphere in a fire is usually of extremely complex composition and, because of the constantly changing conditions the progress of a fire, and the chemical composition (both nature and concentration of materials) varies markedly at different stages of the fire. Also, the characteristics and hazards of one fire may be entirely different from those of another. The chemical composition of the atmosphere and the concentrations of the individual constituents depend on a large number of variable factors; the most important of these include:

- The nature of the materials available for heating or burning.
- Phase of the combustion process.
- The potential for chemical and/or physical interactions between materials present in the fire atmosphere.
- The potential for additive or synergistic toxic effects.
- Temperature.
- Air flow and oxygen availability.

A review of the European and North American literature suggests that some 50-75 per cent of deaths that occur within a few hours of being involved in a fire result from the toxic effects of chemicals in the fire atmosphere. After about 12 h, the contribution of toxic effects of mortalities is considerably less. Over the past few decades the contribution of toxic chemicals to mortalities and non-fatal casualties has increased—for example, in the UK during the period 1955-74 the total number of fire fatalities increased by 70 per cent; those from burns an scalds fluctuated around 400-600 annually, while those attributed to the effects of gas and smoke showed a steady increase (Ballantyne, 1981). The increasing hazard from toxic materials was also shown by consideration of the total incidence of smoke casualties (i.e. fatal and non-fatal): there was a 600 per cent increase over the 19-year period. In the USA there are approximately 600 death annually from fire, with smoke inhalation being responsible for about 80 per cent of the fatalities (Alexaff and Packham, 1984; Kaplan, 1988; Gad, 1990a). Also, the probability of death in increased for the firm victim by smoke inhalation and burns (Zawacki *et al.,* 1977, 1979; Shirani *et al.,* 1986). There are reasonable grounds to believe that the marked increase in smoke and gas casualties in related to the introduction of man-made materials for construction and furnishing. Combustion processes involving polymers result in the generation of variety of lower molecular weight materials which may have significant irritant effects and acute and/or long-term toxicity. The nature and relative amounts to toxic products from combustion of polymers vary both the nature of the polymeric material and the conditions of burning. The range of toxicity possible is reflected in the following examples of typical products from polymer combustion: acetaldehyde, acrolein, phosgene, hydrogen cyanide, carbon monoxide, hydrogeg chloride, and vinyl chloride. It is of practical importance of note that the combustion products of some phosphor-based fire retardants may present toxicological problems (Purser, 1992).

Lethalities resulting from inhalation of chemicals in a fire atmosphere may be due to local chemical injury to the respiratory tract and/ or systemic toxicity following absorption of inhaled materials; the latter may include disturbance of biochemical mechanisms of transport processes, or tissue injury. Non-lethal adverse effects may result from more restricted or less severe local respiratory tract injury or systemic toxicity. It should also be appreciated that inhaled smoke and fumes may contain products of incomplete combustion which continue to release heat following inhalation, resulting in thermal injury to the laryngeal and tracheobronchial mucosa and, with sufficient penetration, to the alveolar epithelium. These thermal injuries will complement any chemically induced respiratory tract injury (Zachria, 1972). Smoke inhalation may lead to pulmonary oedema, in which there is increased permeability of the pulmonary microvasculature (Neimann *et al.,* 1989). Studies of experimentally produced smoke inhalation injury in sheep showed that the primary, and dose-responsive, injury was acute cell membrane damage in the trachea and bronchi leading to oedema, progressive necrotic tracheobronchitis with pseudomem-brane formation, and airways obstruction (Hubbard *et al.*, 1991). Morphological changes occurring in the alveolar epithelium included intracellular oedema (Type I cells), changes in membrane-bound vascuolres (Type II cells), and interstitial oedema.

Although great emphasis has been placed on the acute toxic effects of fire atmospheres, there is also a potential for long-term adverse effects, particularly by repeated exposures. This is considered later in this chapter under a consideration of hazards of firefighting.

Nature and Toxicity of Fire Atmospheres

Thermal decomposition of a material may produce a wide variety of lower molecule species of differing toxicity and irritancy. The number, nature and relative proportions of the products depend on the material burned and the conditions of the combustion process. This may be illustrated by considering the simple burning of wood in an enclosed space. Carbon, hydrogen and sulphur are available as the common combustile elements. In the early phase of burning, sulphur dioxide, water and carbon dioxide are produced, together with some carbon monoxide. As oxygen becomes depleted and burning becomes slower, more carbon monoxide and sulphur dioxide are formed. With further decrease in oxygen availability incomplete combustion occurs and hydrogen, methane, carbon monoxide, and free carbon are produced. In the smouldering phase hydrogen, methane, sulphur dioxide, carbon dioxide, carbon monoxide, free carbon and smoke are all produced. This simple example indicates that as a fire progresses and temperature increases, available oxygen decreases (in enclosed spaces); toxic, irritant and flammable gases are produced and obscuring smoke is formed. Additionally, with combustion of wood, other irritant and toxic materials may be produced; for example, formaldehyde, methanol, acetic acid and other organic irritants (DeKorver, 1976). Even in the apparently simple example of wood, a multiplicity of differing chemicals may be produced; for example, combustion of Douglas fir produced more than 75 discrete chemicals in the smoke. Smoke is usually defined as a complex mixture of airborne solid and liquid particulates and gases produced when a material undergoes thermal decomposition (Kaplan, 1988). Smoke may be obscuring, contain smouldeing particles that can produce thermal injury to the respiratory tract, and contain toxic and irritant materials in gas or vapour form or absorbed on the surface of particulates.

As noted earlier, the widespread introduction of man-made polymeric materials into buildings and furnishings has been associated with a wider spectrum of toxicity than that produced from natural polymers (Alarie, 1985; Gad, 1990a). Products from the combustion of synthetic polymers may have a significant role in morbidity and mortality in fires (Ballantyne, 1981). At low temperatures (up to 400 °C) polymers decompose to give range of complex products; at medium temperatures (400-700 °C) the complexity of products increases and complex organic species may develop at high temperature (>700 °C) complex organic molecules are unstable and decompose (Ballantyne, 1989).

This table shows a few major toxic products but it must be emphasized, that, depending on the condition of combustion, the number of chemical species produced by combustion of a specific polymer may be high. For example polyvinyl chloride yields hydrogen chloride as a principal combustion product but about 75 other organic compounds are generated (Wooley, 1971; Dyer and Each, 1976). Combustion of polyethylene yielded 55 compounds and polypropylene yielded 56 compounds (Mitera and Michal, 1985). With polypropylene, the main thermal degradation products are formaldehyde, acetaldehyde, 2-methylacrolein, acetic acid and acetone (Frostling *et al.*, 1984). Nitrogen-containing polymers may yield hydrogen cyanide and various cyanogens.

Factors Influencing Combustion Products and Their Toxicological Effects

The specific chemical species, and their relative proportions, produced during the combustion processes are dependent on various environmental factors. These factors may, additionally, quantitatively modify the toxic response. The more important factors are summarized below.

Oxygen Availability

The availability of oxygen in the burning area may significantly affect the generation of combustion products. For example, at 500-600 °C polyethylene gives a high acrolein yield with low atmospheric oxygen, and a low acrolein yield when atmospheric oxygen is high (Morikawa, 1976). Clearly this results, at least in part, from proportionately less oxygen being available to maintain vital process where oxygen transport is already compromised by carbon monoxide-induced hypoxia. This is also clearly relevant to practical fire situations, where carbon monoxide is ubiquitous and oxygen depletion common.

Temperature

The temperature in an area of burning or smouldering may significantly influence the products released into the atmosphere. Pyroloysis of polyurethane smoke at 300 °C yields polymeric smoke, but at 800 °C the smoke decomposes to N-containing materials, such as hydrogen cyanide, acetonitrile, acrylonittrile, pyridine and benzonitrile.

Several studies have shown that environmental temperature may influence toxicity. Nomiyama *et al.*, (1980) demonstrated an increase in acute toxicity for various organic solvents, heavy metals and agrochemicals to elevated environmental temperature. Sanders and Endecott (1991) showed, in laboratory rats, that incapacitation occurred earlier when exposure to carbon monoxide was combined with elevated temperature, compared with the effects of carbon monoxide or temperature alone.

Incapacitating Factor in Fires

Incapacitating effects are those that hinder escape from a fire by impairment of physical and/or mental functions. Clearly, obstacles, physical injury and dense smoke are physical factors which may impair mobility and escape. Hypoxia, discussed later, may impair mental functions by a wide range of effects ranging from impairment of judgement to loss of consciousness. Some substances encountered in fire atmospheres may be absorbed and affect CNS function and produce, for example, disturbance of consciousness, abnormalities of coordination, weakness, and decreased reaction and responsiveness times; volatile organic solvents, carbons monoxide and hydrogen cyanide are all examples of materials that produce such effects. These considerations on the effect of hypoxia and absorbed chemicals on behaviour and judgement clearly apply not only to impairment of escape but are also relevant to safe and effective performance by those occupationally involved in firefighting operations.

Many materials of widely varying chemical nature that released in a fire are peripheral sensory irritants. They are thus capable of inducing excess tear production, eye discomfort, and blepharospasm. These ocular effects will clearly result in impairment of vision and thus influence the performance of coordinated tasks and escape from a critical situation.

Hypoxia

Hypoxia is a condition in which there is a physiologically inadequate supply of oxygen to tissues or an impairment of the cellular utilization of oxygen. In the context of a fire, all of the following types of hypoxia may occur.

Hypoxic Hypoxia

This is present where is a decease in the arterial blood PO_2 resulting from inadequate availability of oxygen to blood in pulmonary alveolar capillaries. There is a reduction in the amount of oxygen in arterial blood, but no reduction in PaO_2. This may be a consequence depletion of atmospheric oxygen in the inspired air, airways obstruction, lung injury sufficient to reduce diffusing capacity, low tidal volume, or increased dead space.

Anaemic Hypoxia

This is present when there is a decreased oxygen transporting capacity of the blood, as, for example, a reduced circulating erythrocyte mass. In a fire, anaemic hypoxia may occur from reduced haemoglobin oxygen binding sites which is frequently a result of carboxyhaemoglobin formation or the induction of methaemoglo-binaemia.

Cytotoxic Hypoxia

This is a systemic effect where there is interference with the utilization of oxygen by cells. A classic examples is that of inhibition of cellular cytochrome oxidase activity by cyanide. Hypoxia is a broad term referring to inadequate tissue supply or utilization of oxygen for any reason; hypoxaemia refers only to decreased carriage of oxygen in arterial blood (as in hypoxic and anaemic hypoxia). Although tissue oxygen supply is decreased in hypoxaemia, significant damage does not occur until arterial oxygen saturation falls to about 50 per cent and PaO_2 falls to about 30 mm Hg (Campbell *et al.*, 1984).

If of sufficient degree, hypoxia may result in death. Lesser degrees of hypoxia, however, are highly significant in fires because of the following possibilities.

- The development, sometimes insidious of neurological abnormalities. These may include impaired coordination, impaired judgement, disturbance of consciousness ranging from drowsiness to coma and disorientation (Autian, 1976; Ganong, 1977). All these can clearly produce variable degrees of mental and/or physical incapacitation.
- Hypoxia may increase chemoreceptor activity, leading

to an increase in the rate and depth of breathing. This could result in enhanced inhalation exposure to toxic materials in sinspried air.

- As mentioned earlier, hypoxia may enhance the toxicity of some materials.

Examples of Common Materials in Fire Atmospheres

Carbon monoxide is a major and ubiquitoru component of fire atmospheres, often at potentially lethal concentrations (Jankovic et al., 1991). Barnard (1979) measured carbon monoxide concentrations in 25 Los Angeles fires and found that in 12 per cent of fires the peak carbon monoxide was less than 100 ppm. in 40 per cent peak values were in range 501-1000 ppm, 25 per cent in the range 500-1000 ppm, and 23 per cent in than 1000 ppm; the highest concentration measured was 3000 ppm. A major factor in the toxicity of carbon monoxide is generally considered to be related to its high affinity for haemoglobin, being about 250 times that of oxygen. A sufficient exposure to carbon monoxide is the fact that the presence of carboxyhaemoglobin (COHb) cause a shift-to-the-left of the oxygen-haemoglobin dissociation curve. As a consequence there is increased affinity of haemoglobin for oxygen, and thus at any given PO_2 the release of oxygen will be reduced compared with conditions where COHb is not present (Ayres et al., 1973). Also, carbon monoxide inhibits cytochrome a_3; this will be a function of plasma carbon monoxide (Goldbaum et al., 1976; Goldbaum, 1977).

Interpretation of COHb values, particularly at lower concentrations, needs to be undertaken carefully because of the influence of environment (rural or urban) factors, and cigarette smoking on COHb concentrations (Ballantyne, 1981). Also, if dicloromethane is present, this may be endogenously converted to carbon monoxide (Hathaway *et al.*, 1991). Additionally, if analysis for COHb is not performed promptly in appropriately stored containers, analytica arteface losses may occur (Chance *et al.*, 1986; Levin *et al.*,

1990). The majority of individuals exposed to fire atmospheres will have elevated concentrations of COHb, the degree of which depends on the exposure time and exposure concentration. Low concentrations of COHb may indicate rapid death from trauma or extensive burning (Levin *et al.*, 1990; Mayes, 1990; Mayes, 1991; Mayes *et al.*, 1992). When death is solely from carbon monoxide poisoning (for example coal gas poisoning) the COHb concentrations stated to be compatible with death from acute carbon monoxide poisoning are usually in the range 50-60 per cent. COHb concentrations [COHb] measured in fire victims may show a wide spectrum of values, some compatible with death from carbon monoxide poisoning, others significantly lower. For example, Harland and Wooley (1979) in a sample of 90 fire deaths found [COHb] of more than 50 per cent in half the cases; those above 50 per cent had a mean value of 67 per cent and those below a mean of 18 per cent. In interpreting lower concentrations of COHb in fatal cases; it should be remembered that hypoxia may enhance the toxicity of carbon monoxide, and that carbon monoxide toxicity may be an interactive factor in the presence of other toxic substance and physical and thermal trauma. Patterns of [COHb] found in differing fires may reflect the circumstance of an individual specific fire. For example, in the MGM Grand Hotel fire 51.3 per cent of victims had [COHb] of more than 50 per cent; in this fire most of the victims were found in areas remote from the conflagration (Birky *et al.*, 1985). In contrast, in the DuPont Plaza Hotel fire in Puerto Rico, 80-85 per cent of the victims had [COHb] of less than 50 per cent; in this fire the majority of victims were burned and bound in the area of the fire (Levin *et al.*, 1990).

Exposure to sublethal concentrations of carbon monoxide may result in various potentially adverse health effects. Of notable importance are neurological and behavioural effects which could hinder the performances of skilled tasks or the recognition of, and escape from, a critical situation. These includes headache, dizziness, disturbance of vision, confusion, difficulties in coordination, decreased reaction time, and drowsiness (Stewart, 1974; Zarem *et al.*, 1973). Additionally, acute exposure to carbon monoxide may produce cardiac arrythmias, myocardial damage, and circulatory failure (Stewart, 1974). Also, there may be aggravation of exercise-induced angina, decreased exercise tolerance, depression of the S-T segment in the ECG, and increased vulnerability to ventricular fibrillation (Anderson *et al.*, 1973; Aronow, 1976; De Bias *et al.*, 1976).

The human foetus is particularly sensitive to carbon monoxide because of several differences from the adult. Under steady-state conditions foetal [COHb] is around 10-15 per cent greater than the corresponding maternal blood [COBh]. Additionally, the partial pressure of oxygen in foetal blood is lower, at 20-30 mmHg, compared with the adult value of 100 mmHG (Longo, 1976, 1977; McDiarmid *et al.*, 1991). Furthermore, the fetal oxygen-haemoglobin dissociation curve lies to the left to the adult curve, resulting in greater tissue hopoxia to equivalent COHb concentrations. It is also considered that the foetal half-life of elimination of carbon monoxide is longer than in mother (Margulies, 1986). Acute exposure to carbon monoxide concentrations that are non-lethal to the mother have been associated with foetal loss (Muller and Graham, 1955; Goldstein, 1965), or permanent neurological sequelae in the foetus (Cramer, 1982). These factors need to be considered in relation to pregnant women exposed to fire atmospheres, and the employment of women of childbearing age in the fire services.

Hydrogen Cyanide

Any material containing carbon and nitrogen will liberate hydrogen cyanide (HCN) under appropriate combustion conditions. In addition, various cyanogens may be produced such as acrylonitrile, acetonitrile, adiponitrile, benzonitrile and propionitrile. Cyanogen has also been detected in the blood of fire victims. Polymeric materials are particularly notable source of HCN; for example, nylon (Purser an Wooley, 1983), polyacrylonitrile (Bertol *et al.*, 1983), polyurethanes. Urea formaldehyde (Paabo *et al.*,1979) and melamine. Although some studies show that the evolution of HCN is proportional to the nitrogen content of polymeric materials (Morikawa, 1978), this is not a universal finding. Bertol *et al.* (1983) found that proportionately more HCN (1500 ppm) was evolved from polyacrylonitrile (19.0 per cent elemental nitrogen) than from wool (200 ppm; 14.3 per cent elemental nitrogen). Also, Urhas and Kullik (1977) found that with pyrolysis temperature in the range of 625-925 °C, the yield of HCN was inversely related to the nitrogen content of three fibres. Both temperature and oxygen availability influence the yield of HCN from a nitrogen-containing material.

In oxidizing atmospheres, HCN is evolved at lower temperatures and as temperature increases so does HCN liberation, up to maximum, andthen decrease with further in temperature; a secondary rise in HCN may occur at even higher temperatures. Polyester and polyether flexible urethane foams decompose at relatively low temperature (200-300 °C) in inert atmospheres to produce a yellow smoke which is stable up to 800 °C; however, over the range of 800-1000°C there is decomposition yielding HCN, acetonitrile, benzonitrile and pyridine as the major nitrogen-containing products (Wooley, 1972). These and many other studies indicate that the evolution of HCN varies with temperature, oxygen availability, the chemical nature of the nitrogen-containing material, and the burning time. Although these variables will differ at any given time, practical estimates for HCN generation have ben made. For example, Morikawa (1978) calculated that if nylon is burned at 950 °C under restricted air conditions, then only 1.5 g is necessary to raise the HCN concentration to around 135 ppm in a 1 m^3 space. Extrapolating data from combustion studies, Bertol *et al.*, (1983) calculated that a toxic concentration of HCN could be developed in an average-sized room by the burning of 2 kg polyacrylonitrile.

As with animal studies, there is a wealth of information suggesting that humans exposed to combustion products have absorbed cyanide. The first detailed description of cyanide in the blood of fire victims was given by Wetherell (1966) who found cyanide in the blood of 39 to 53 individuals dying in fires; the average concentration was 0.65 μg ml^{-1} (range 0.17-2.20 μg ml^{-1}). Other representative studies are as follows. Hart *et al.* (1985) described five subjects with smoke inhalation who were comatose on admission to hospital: blood cyanide ranged from 0.35 to 3.9 μg ml^{-1} (average 1.62 μg m^{-1}). The subject with the highest blood cyanide died 4 days after admission. In postcrash aeroplane fires, Mohler (1975) reported blood cyanide in victims in the range of 0.01-3.9 μg ml^{-1}. In some case, increased cyanide concentrations clearly indicate death from acute cyanide poisoning; for example. Tscuhiay (1977) described two persons found dead after a fire involving a polyurethane matters with blood cyanide concentrations of 7.2 and 23.0 μg ml^{-1}, respectively.

Exposure to HCN vapour released in a fire can lead to muscle weakness, difficulty in coordination, physical incapacitation, a confusional state, and partial or complete loss of consciousness. This clearly will impede escape from the area of a fire. The high concentration of cyanide measured in fire casualties has raised the question of the use of cyanide antidotes in cases of severe smoke inhalation (Daunderer, 1979; Hart *et al.,* 1985). HCN as a product of combustion, and its significance, has been reviewed by Ballantyne (1987).

Toxic Inter-Relationships Between Fire Gas Components

As has been repeatedly stressed, the fire atmosphere is continually varying complex of numberous chemicals of differing chemical structure and differing toxicity. The acute and long-term hazards of many, but not all, individual components are known to varying extends. The influence of interactive factors on known toxicity and the additional interactive toxicity is, however, poorly understood. Nevertheless, studies have been conducted for a few binary chemical systems. Several illustrative example are given below, which demonstrate that even with such simple binary systems the hazard may vary according to the relative proportion of the components.

Hydrogen Cyanide-Carbon Monoxide

As CO and HCN coexist in a fire, this is a highly practical consideration, and has been discussed in detail by Ballantyne (1987). The approaches have been variable and have included mortality studies, measurements of blood cyanide and COHb, and assessment of physiological functions. Moss *et al.* (1951) found that simultaneous exposure to CO (2000 ppm) and HCN (10-20 ppm), both at individually sublethal concentrations, caused death, Smith *et al.* (1976) found that the times to death for rats exposed to an atmosphere containing 450 ppm HCN and 13500 ppm CO (3.7 ± 0.4 min; mean ± SD) were slightly longer than for corresponding concentrations of HCN along (10.9 + 2.0 min; mean ± SD) or CO alone (5.8 ± 1.2 min; mean ± SD). Norris *et al.* (1986) investigated the effect of a 3-min inhalation exposure of mice to CO (0.63-0.66 per cent) in the lethal toxicity of intraperitoneal KCN (4-9 mg kg^{-1}). A significantly lower LD_{50} for KCN (6.51; 6.04-7.00 mg kg^{-1}; mean with 95% CL) was found in Cooperated animals than in air-alone controls (7.0; 7.36-8.45 mg kg^{-1}; mean with 95% CL). In further studies they found evidence for a synergism between CO and KCN. The authors suggested that this may have been the result of augmentation of the inhibition of cytochrome oxidase in the CNS. Pitt *et al.,* (1979) investigated the effects of CO and HCN on cerebral circulation and metabolism in the dog. When given together, CO and HCN increased cerebral blood flow in an additive manner; however, a significant decrease the cerebral oxygen consumption occurred with combined exposure to CO and HCN, neither of which alone had an effect. Balantyne (1984, 1987) investigated the effects of differing proportions of HCN and CO in the atmosphere on lethal toxicity and on blood cyanide and COHb concentrations, and determined that the contribution of either substance to toxicity depends in their absolute and relative atmospheric concentrations. Thus, when there was a marked excess of CO, the presence of HCN lowered the lethal inhalation dosage for CO by a less than additive toxicity; i.e. HCN physiologically potentiated (by hyperventilation) the toxicity of CO. When there was excess CO with respect to HCN, but not sufficient to produce a clear biochemical evidence of death from CO, then the blood picture indicated death not primarily from either CO or HCN. In these circumstances, because of the less than additive toxicity, it is likely that both are acting at a common target site, probably cytiochrome oxidase. When CO and HCN are present in equal mass proportions, biochemical evidence indicates that death results from acute cyanide poisoning.

Carbon Monoxide-Carbon Dioxide

Nelson *et al.* (1978) found the 30-min lethal concentration of CO to rats was 6000 ppm, which was decreased to 2560 ppm in the presence of 1.44 per cent CO_2. Redkey and Collison (1979) found more rapid times to death in rats exposed to 6000 ppm CO with 4.5 per cent CO_2 (16.8 ± 0.6 min) compared with 6000 ppm alone. Levin *et al.* (1989), in detailed studies, found that above a certain concentration of CO (4100 ppm) some rats will die, and adding CO_2 has no influence. Below 2500 ppm CO the addition of CO_2 (up to 17.7 per cent) is not sufficient to produce mortality. However, with a CO concentrations range of 2500-4100 ppm (which produces few moralities *per se*) CO_2 (more than 1.5 per cent) will produce a higher level of mortality. They noted that CO and CO_2 act together by (1) increasing the rate of COHb formation, (2) producing a severe acidosis which was greater than the metabolic acidosis from CO alone or respiratory acidosis from CO_2 alone, and (3) prolonging the recovery period from acidosis.

Investigation of The Toxicological Hazards of Fires

Investigation into, and assessment of, potential adverse health effects from the products of combustion are complex exercises because of the multiplicity of thermolysis products and the variability of factors affecting the qualitative and quantitative nature of the products and the biological responses to them. Therefore, in respect of most practical situations it is possible only to give an overview of the products likely to be present under given conditions of thermolysis, and a qualitative assessment of hazards. Although detailed studies have been carried out on some binary systems, allowing quantitative assessments for interactions to be made, the majority of studies have been conducted to overall combustion products. An outline of the various approaches to investigating toxicological hazards from fires is given below; details can be found in Gad (1990b) and Kaplan (1988).

Physicochemical Studies on Thermolysis Products

These laboratory studies are concerned with the analytical determination of the chemical nature and relative proportions of substances produced by thermolysis of materials under differing conditions. Ideally, the analyses should be conducted under the following conditions: simple heating, complete combustion, oxidative pyrolysis, and anaerobic pyrolysis. It is thus necessary to subject materials to a range of temperatures in atmospheres of differing oxygen content, with the resultant effluent being analyzed by appropriate instrumental procedures. In some instances, highly toxic materials may be generated over a narrow temperature range, and if a differential temperature study is not performed this may be missed. In addition to the influence of temperature and oxygen availability on the materials generated from combustion, it is important to study the nature of the materials generated as a function of time period in the combustion phase because the pattern may change appreciably.

From a knowledge of the nature of the materials generated, under different conditions of combustion, it may be possible to give a hazard pattern for a given material providing that adequate information on toxicology is available. In some cases a major hazardous material may be identified from a large number of analytically detected substances produced by combustion of a specific material. With polyvinyl chloride (PVC) about 75 organic products have been detected on thermal decomposition, most being aliphatic or aromatic hydrocarbons (Wooley, 1971). However, a major product which begins to be liberated at 200-300 °C is hydrogen chloride, and it is estimated that 1 kg of PVC may yield about 400 g of hydrogen chloride on complete combustion. Hydrogen chloride causes sensory irritation of the eyes and respiratory tract, and in sufficient concentrations may cause inflammatory lesions in the respiratory tract. PVC combustion is recognized as a major hazard in fires involving modern buildings.

The small-scale laboratory tests yield useful, though often preliminary, information on the nature of combustion products generated from specific material under defined conditions and allow a qualitative assessment of the hazards that may be encountered for a specific material in a fire. The majority of fires, however, involve the burning of multiplicity of materials including structural and furnishing components. In an attempt to obtain more reliable information it may be desirable to undertake large-scale experimental fires with appropriate instrumentation. Such tests are likely to be expensive and require careful planning, specifically with regard to sampling and analysis of the atmosphere. Guidance on the design of large-scale tests will clearly be obtained from preliminary small-scale laboratory combustion product studies.

Animal Exposure Studies

In the strictly physicohemical analytical approach to defining the nature and relative proportions of combustion products generated from specific materials, the likely hazard of the effluent smoke is determined by attempting to predict the probable combined toxicity of the constituents in the smoke from a knowledge of their individual toxicities. Such an approach may produce misleading predictions because there is the possibility of chemical and toxicological interactions, including synergism. Attempt have therefore been made to determine the toxicity of smokes from specific material by exposing animals to the products of thermolysis and monitoring for adverse effects by standard and special procedures. Such tests readily tend themselves to observations on irritancy and acute toxicity. Irritancy will give an index of potentially harassing and in capacitating properties of effluent, smoke from the material, and the acute toxicity an indication of lethal potential or obvious non-lethal adverse effects such as lung damage, or neurobehavioural abnormalities. Such tests are frequently carried out with the smoke being generated under differing conditions of atmospheric oxygen content and thermolysis temperature. For comparative purposes the findings are frequently referred to tests from the burning of a standard material, usually wood. Although such tests give useful information in themselves, they are particularly valuable when viewed in the light of studies on the analysis of combustion products generated under similar conditions. Thus, when interpreting laboratory data in an attempt to define possible hazards from combustion products of materials it is highly desirable to have information on both the nature and relative proportions of combustion products and on their effects on experimental animals exposed to combustion products generated under similar conditions. Where appropriate facilities and expertise exists it is possible to combine analytical studies with animal exposure tests. Also, animal exposures have been performed in large-scale fire tests.

Problems may be encountered in defining the presence of novel or highly toxic materials for several reasons; first because of the multiplicity of materials generated there may be limitations in analytical capability and second, the toxicology of some materials generated may be unknown. However, animal studies may draw attention to the presence of highly toxic or unsuspected, materials in a test atmosphere. This may be illustrated by investigations on a fire-retarded polyurethane foam. The producers from non-flaming combustion of a trimethylol-propane-based rigid urethane foam fire retarded with an organophosphate, *O, O*-diethyl-*N, N*-Bis (2-hydroxyethyl)-aminomethhly phosphonate, were found to produce grand mal seizures in rats; similar effects were not observed when the foam was not fire retarded (Petajan *et al.,* 1974). Subsequent chemical analysis revealed the presence of 4-ethyl-1-phospha-2,6,7-trixabicyclo [2,2,2] octane-1-oxide in the smoke (Voorhees *et al.,* 1975). This is a material of high acute toxicity (Kimmerle, 1976). Further work demonstrated no unusual toxicity when the flame-retarded polyurethane foam was either gradually or rapidly pyrolyzed to 800 °C in the absence of air; however, convulsions were observed when the material was flash pyrolyzed in the presence of air flow (Hilado and Schneider, 1977). See Purser (1992) for a discussion of caged bicyclophosphorus esters in combustion processes.

Combustion Toxicity Apparatus

Several apparatuses are currently available: the DIN 53-436 (a German standard), the radiant furnace (an ASTM draft standard), and the University of Pittsburgh furnace (an ASTM draft standard and legislated in the State of New York). The selection of the apparatus will depend on the combustion conditions that are to be simulated. Some possible combustion conditions are smouldering, flaming, preflashover and post-flashover. These apparatuses have different capabilities for simulating these combustion conditions.

The DIN 53-438

The combustion device is moving annual furnace encircling a quartz tube containing the test specimen. The intent of this design is to generate a consistent combustion environment for the time course of the experiment even though the animal exposure is dynamic. The furnace temperature is a fixed value during the experiment but that value can range between 100 and 900 °C. The animals are rats, and the exposure is head only. After the exposure, the animal are retained for a 2-week postexposure period. Selection of the temperature can determine the combustion of conditions of the test specimen for on-flaming or flaming mode.

The Radiant Furnace

The combustion device is a set of four quartz lamps designed to subject the test specimen to a heat flux density ranging from 2 to 7 kW m^{-2}. The animal exposure to the combustion products is static. The animals are rats, and the exposure is head only. The rats are observed for 2 weeks after exposure. The combustion conditions can be selected by changing the heat flux density and implementing the use of a piloted ignition source. Thus, non-flaming and flaming conditions can be investigated. The LCt_{50} (medium lethal concentration × time of exposure) value is expressed as (mg min 1 ^{1}). The methodology is currently an ASTM draft standard.

The University of Pittsburgh

The combustion device is basically a muffle furnace. The test specimen is subjected to a ramping temperature of 20 °C per min. The animal exposure to the combustion products is dynamic. The animals are mice, and the exposure is lead only. After the test specimen has lost 1 per cent of its initial weight the combustion products are presented to the animals. The exposure period is ended 30 min later. For 10 min after the exposure period the animals are observed. The combustion conditions are the same for all the test specimens. However, the test specimen can react differently to those conditions, thereby combusting in a non-flaming or flaming mode. The critical variable appears to be the weight of the specimen. The smaller weight specimens will not necessarily spontaneously flame, while larger weight specimens many spontaneously fame. Thus, more than one LC_{50} value can be obtained for a test substance (Norris, 1990).

The LC_{50} value is expressed as grams. This is the weight of the test specimen placed in the furnace which is calculated to kill 50 per cent of the animals. The State of New York legislated that certain building products be tested by this procedure and those results field with the state before the products could be sold. New York City also used this test for pas/fail criteria for some building materials. The methodology is currently an ASTM draft standard.

Studies on Exposed Human Population

Valuable and unique information may be obtain about the adverse effects of exposure to fire atmospheres, and on the possible long-term hazards of recurrent exposures to fires, by appropriate studies on the victims of fires and on firefighters. Major sources of information have been derived from post-morterm examination of fire victims; clinical, radiological and clinical chemistry examination of non-lethal fire victims; and routine medical examination and special epidemiological studies of firefighters. In the context of defining requirement for respiratory and other protective equipment by firefighters based on the medical and epidemiological data, shor-term repeated and chronic exposure situations as well as acute exposures all require consideration.

Toxic Hazard and Hazard Analysis

In 1986 the US National Institute of Building Sciences initiated a programme to develop to develop a performance toxicity test to characterize building products. This performance test was developed so that it incorporated additional fire parameters, such as LC_{50} value, time to ignition, and mass loss rate. The concern was that regulation of products was to occur based solely on the LC_{50} values. As a hazard analysis was not available, this was viewed as an interim step until the complete hazard analysis could be established (Norris, 1988). The methodology is currently an ASTM draft standard.

The direction for utilization of combustion toxicity data

has been to include them in hazard analysis. These analysis include other fire performance parameters, such as time to ignition, flame spread, heat release rate, etc. The fire scenario is also a part of these analysis. The US National Institute of Standards and Technology has developed a hazard analysis called HAZARD 1 Fire Hazard Assessment Method (Bukowski *et al,* 1989).

Chemical Hazards to Firefighters

Firefighting is one of the most hazardous of professions, having an associated high level of morbidity and mortality, with the most important health concerns being as follows.

(1) *Trauma:* notably from falling objects, in rescue situations, and during close-in firefighting.
(2) *Thermal:* primary burns to the skin and respiratory tract, and heat stress. The latter is a function of environmental temperature, insulating properties of protective clothing, and endogenous heat production from severe physical exertion compounded by the additional weight of equipment such as self-contained breathing apparatus.
(3) *Ergonomic:* the high energy costs of firefighting may clearly be interrelated with, and compounded by other health concerns.
(4) *Psychological:* these are multiple in nature and include the thought of personal security, victim rescue and loss, emotional scenes, and heavy social responsibility (Guidotti and Clough, 1992).
(5) *Toxic chemicals:* sequential exposure to smoke and chemicals, often at high concentrations, which are known or suspect of producing acute and/or long-term health problems. An outline of this aspect of health concern is presented below; details are available from Guidotti and Clough (1992).

Firefighters are recurrently exposed to a large variety of materials that may cause acute, cumulative, and/or chronic health problems; typical examples are carbon monoxide, hydrogen cyanide, sulphur dioxide, hydrogen chloride, phosgene, isocyanates, oxides of nitrogen, acrolein, acetaldehyde, asbestos, polycylic aromatic hydrocarbons and benzene. That such materials may be absorbed has been suggested buy several studies; for example, that firefighters absorb HCN is indicated by increased serum thiocyanate concentrations (Levine and Radford, 1978). As expected, several studies have demonstrated that firefighters have increased blood COHb concentrations. Sammons and Coleman (1974) found a significant difference in BOHb concentrations between non-smoking firemen (mean 5.0 per cent, range 2.5-13.9 per cent) and non-smoking controls (mean 2.3 per cent, range 1.0-11.7 per cent). Similarly, Radford and Levine (1976) found increased COHb concentrations in firemen after fighting a fire (4.53 per cent) compared with unexposed controlled (2.17 per cent). Increased COHb concentrations were also found after firefighting by Loke *et al.,* (1970) and Levy *et al.,* (1976).

Respiratory Disease

Several studies have shown that exposure to a fire atmosphere produces acute changes in pulmonary function and may be a factor in the development of chronic lung dysfunction. Musk *et al.* (1979) studied acute changes in firefighters during routine duties and found an average decrease of FEV_1 (forced expiratory volume in 1 s) of 0.05 1 which was related to subjectively assessed smoke exposure; decreases in FEV_1 of 0.1 1 or more were found in 30 per cent of cases. Brandt-Rauf *et al.* (1989) found that for firefighters not wearing respiratory protective equipment, there were statistically significant postfire decrements in FEV_1 and FVC (forced vital capacity). Pre-and postfire average FEV_1 values respectively 3.80 1 and 3.61 1, and FVC values 5.03 1 and 4.81 1 (n = 14).

For cumulative effects, Peabody (1977) reported a decrease in pulmonary function for San Diego firefighters which was significantly greater than that of the general population. Peters *et al.* (1974), over a 2-year period, found that the rate of decline in pulmonary function, measured by FVC and FEV_1, was twice the expected rate; these changes were significantly related to frequency of exposure. A raised risk for emphysema was found in a mortality study by Demers *et al.* (1992). The importance of respiratory protective equipment was shown in a study by Tepper *et al.* (1991) who reevaluated 632 Baltimore city firemen 6-10 years after baseline measurements, and found that in those who never wore a mask there was a 1.7 times greater decline than in mask wearers.

Cardiovascular Disease

Some epidemiological studies do not shown an excess of cardiovascular disease among firemen (Beaumont *et al.*, 1991; Demers *et al.*, 1992). Summarizing the available evidence, Guidotti (1992) states that population-based mortality and disability surveillance studies suggest a relatively small but significant excess of disability, but not mortality, for non-maligant cardiovascular disease for firefighters. More targeted cohort and case-control studies do not support such an excess, but suggest a strong healthy worker effect. However, some studies suggest an excess of coronary artery disease (Musk *et al.*, 1978).

Reproductive Hazards

Many of the chemicals that are found in a fire atmosphere have been associated with potential adverse reproductive effects (McDiarmid *et al.*, 1991). In spite of this, little edidemiological evidence is available on the reproductive hazards of fire fighting. One study has indicated a possible excess of birth defects in children of firefighters (Olshan *et al.*, 1990). Also, it has been noted that peak carbon monoxide concentrations measured in fires could be immediately dangerous to an unprotected woman firefighter and her foetus (McDiarmid *et al.*, 1991). There is a clear need for further investigation into the reproductive hazards of firefighting.

Carninogenic Hazards

Several known or suspect carcinogens are present, to variable extents, in fire atmospheres; for example, ploycylic aromatic hydrocarbons, acrylonitrile, vinyl chloride asbestos, formal-dehyde and PCBs. There are some inconsistencies between various studies on the possible excess of cancers in firefighters. Biological monitoring for genotoxic effects, including sister chromatid exchanges and polycylic aromatic hydrocarbon-DNA adducts in peripheral blood, suggests a potential for carcinogenic effects (Liou *et al.,* 1989). Particular sites for neoplasms, possibly occupationally related to firefighting, are buccal and pharyngeal (Mastromatteo, 1974), oesophageal (Beaumont *et al.,* 1991), colonorectal (Guidotti and Clough, 1992), brain (Howe and Burch, 1990; Demers *et al.,* 1992), lymphatic and leukaemic (Demers *et al.,* 1992). Documentation for an association between lung cancer and occupational exposures is inconsistent. A Danish study (Hansen, 1990) reported an SMR of 317 for older firefighters, but studies from San Francisco (Beaumont *et al.,* 1991) and Buffalo (Vena and Fielder, 1987) showed no excess. Cigarette smoking is a clear confounding factor (Liou *et al.,* 1989), although according to one study the incidence of smoking among firemen is not excessive compared with other occupations (Gerace, 1990). The excesses of certain cancers may be the result of interaction of several factors; for example, toxic substances, alcohol and smoking (Beaumont *et al.,* 1991). Ford *et al.,* 1992) suggest that the immunological detection of serum β-transforming growth factor-related proteins may be a possible biomarker for monitoring firefighters for potential development of cancer.

8

Toxicology of the Adrenal, Thyroid and Endocrine Pancreas

Introduction

There are many target organs in the endocrine system that are sensitive to chemical and drug insult (Thomas and Keenan, 1986). Both the male and the female reproductive systems are vulnerable to chemically induced changes. Likewise, the foetus and the neonates can be affected by chemicals and drugs (Thomas 1989). Gonadal to toxicities and teratogenesis are important aspects of endocrine aberrations brought about by either chemicals or drugs (Thomas and Ballantyne, 1990). Reproductive toxicology and development toxicology certainly can involved the endocrine system. However, there are other non-global target organs in the endocrine system that can be affected by drugs and chemicals.

The thyroid gland, the adrenal gland and the pancreas can each be affected by various drugs and chemicals (Thomas *et al.*, 1985). In the case of the thyroid and adrenal glands, drugs, and synthetic steroids can interface with their internal secretions either by affecting the glands directly or by interfering with trophic hormone secretion at the level of the adenohypophysis. Because numerous drugs and related factors can affect the secretion and/or release of adenohypophyseal hormones, it is important to be aware of such factors or condition when attempting clinically to assess piiuitary function. With the advent of radioimmunoassays (RIA) it is now possible to assess the blood levels of most trophic hormones. Drug-induced alterations of pituitary function tests can lead to misinterpretations and therapeutic misadventure. Indeed, the results of pituitary function can be altered by many endogenous and exogenous agents (Thomas *et al.,* 1989).

It is estimated that nearly 90 per cent of all endocrine toxicities appear in the adrenal gland, the test and the thyroid gland. Some endocrine organs appear to be more sensitive to toxic agents, and this often lead to multiple disruptions in the hormonal balance of organism. It is not uncommon for chemically induced changes in gonadal function to affect the activity of the thyroid gland. Chemically induced changes in sex steroids can affect pancreatic secretion of insulin. Chemically induced stress leading to an increased secretion of glucocorticoids can also affect insulin secretion, but more importantly can affect adrenocorticotropin (ACTH) levels and hence alter the pituitaryadrenal axis.

The thalidomide tragedy of the 1960s led to the formulation of toxicological testing guidelines for the field of teratology. Thereafter, selected protocol for reproductive and development toxicology tests were instituted. Generally, test requirements have not been imposed for other endocrine organs. Chemically induced changes in the endocrine system can be purposeful. For example, synthetic steroids can effectively suppress pituitary gonadotropins, thereby affording millions of women with a chemical method of birth control. The chemical suppression of excessive endogenous hormone secretion also can be therapeutically achieved in he adrenal and thyroid glands.

Pituitary

A knowledge of hormonal feedback systems is of value

in attempting to predict the effect(s) of potentially toxic agents on a particular endocrine target organ (Thomas and Keenan, 1986). Although the measurement of specific hormone levels might not be possible for all general toxicological screenings of substances, some bioassays and microscopic techniques may yield useful information. For example, a slowing in animal growth rates, in most instances caused by diminished nutritional intake, can result from the pression of pituitary growth hormone (GH) secretion. Similarly, a decrease in adrenal weights following the administration of certain chemicals can be caused by an interference with pituitary ACTH.

Generally, chemically induced changes that affect pituitary-target organ relationship seldom manifest themselves after a single administration of a toxic agent. Rather, compounds that have the potential to exert deleterious effects on the endocrine system ordinarily require longer durations of exposure and repeated administrations. While chemically induced stress can provoke a rapid response in catecholamine secretion and an outpouring of glucocorticoids, other hormonal changes would ordinarily not be so immediate. Agents causing the induction of hepatic microsomal enzyme systems that affect hormone metabolism usually require upwards of a week before hormone changes in the endocrine systems.

It is important to understand some of the more basic or classical hormonal relationships between the adenohypophysis and the respective endocrine target organs. Chemicals, including certain classes of therapeutically effective drugs, can interfere with the release of trophic hormones or can interfere with their synthesis (Thomas and Keenan, 1986). Still other toxic agents inhibitory actions on the biosynthesis of target organ hormone secretions. Thus, there are several sites of actions of different chemicals on the adenohypophyseal-target organ feedback systems.

Depending on the particular chemical, the sites of action may differ in their sensitivity to toxic agents. Target organs such as the gonads are sensitive to toxic substances because rapidly dividing cells are often vulnerable to chemical destruction. Environmental stresses can affect the secretory activity of certain of the hypothalamic-releasing hormones, and hence alter pituitary-target organ relationships. Sometimes toxic agents can bind to circulating blood proteins and alter the ratio of free and bound forms of target organ hormones. Such changes in binding canal so modify the pituitary-target hormone relationship.

Adenohypophysis

As the trophic hormones are either protein or glycoprotein in chemical composition, they cannot be measured by standard spectrophotometric procedures. These hormones must either be bioassayed or measured by using RIA (Thomas *et al.,* 1989). Bioassays were useful for certain of the adenohypophyseal hormones but such tests have been replaced by newer and more sensitive RIA. Bioassays, however, might be employed where there is only a secondary interest in determining whether a particular toxicological agent is affecting trophic hormone levels. Sometimes a target organ that is known to be directly influenced by a particular trophic hormone can examined, and provide general insights into the nature of the chemically induced alterations in the endocrine system. Despite the more complex and involved RIA methodologies, they are of immense value for measuring different hormones. RIA represents an analytical approach of great sensitivity, and such techniques have been applied to well over 200 biological substances, many of which cannot be assayed by other techniques. Unlike bioassays that often require large amounts of tissue (or blood), the greater sensitivity of the RIA can be achieved with the very small samples of biological fluids.

Some hormone can be measured by competitive assays either by utilizing an immune system or a non-immune system. In the immune system assay the antibody acts as the binding protein (e.g. insulin, ACTH), whereas in the non-immune assays system the binding the reagent if often a naturally-occurring protein with a high affinity for the hormone being measured (e.g. cortisol, thyroxine). Monoclonal antibodies are also used in the measurement of various hormones.

The concept of radioassays, whether the binding protein is an antibody or a naturally occurring protein with a high affinity for the hormone to be measured, is the same. Basically, the binding sites are saturated with a radioactive form of the hormone and, subsequently, incubated with the non-radioactive form of the hormone that is to be measured. Competition occurs between the radioactive and the non-radioactive form of the hormone. The ratio of antibody-bound to free (unbound) radioactive hormone is reduced as the concentration of non-radioactive hormone is increased. By using solutions containing known amounts of hormone, a standard curve and be constructed, thus providing a sensitive competitive binding assay for a particular hormone. Other immunoassasys can likewise be used.

Measurement of Anterior Pituitary Hormones

Modulation of adrenocortical growth and secretory activity is by ACTH. ACTH exerts a number of physiological actions, including maintenance of the adrenal gland and stimulation of adrenal gland and stimulation of adrenal cortical steroid secretion. ACTH can cause depletion of adrenal gland ascorbic acid.

There are several pathological states that can alter ACTH secretion. Furthermore, stress induced from any one of a variety of environmental or chemicals stimuli can cause a rapid elevation in ACTH blood levels. There is a diurnal rhythm for the secretion of corticosteroids.

Several methods are available for measuring ACTH but most assays resort to assessing adrenal gland parameters (Thomas *et al.,* 1989). Certainly, the gravimetric assay to adrenal glands represent one for the simplest methods for indirectly evaluating ACTH activity. In hypophysectomized animals (e.g. rats), ACTH injections can maintain the weight of the adrenal glands. ACTH stimulates increases in plasma cortisol and corticosterone and elevates urinary 17-hydroxycorticosteroids and 17-ketosteroids, which can be used as an index of adrenal cortex function. ACTH causes involution of the thymus gland, deposition of hepatic glycogen, and leads to a decrease in circulating eosinophils in hypophysectomized rodents. These latter ACTH-induced changes in these biological parameters have also been used to assess ACTH activity.

Radioligand-receptor assays and other immuno-assays have been developed for ACTH. These RIA are very sensitive but can represent a considerable investment of time and expense for routine toxicological assessment of pituitaryad-renal axis.

Thyroid-Stimulating Hormone (TSH)

Thyroid-stimulating hormone (TSH) is a glycoprotein capable of stimulating the growth and proliferation of cells of the thyroid gland. TSH can produce a number of biochemical and histological changes in the thyroid gland. TSH assays have employed the uptake of ^{32}P in the thyroid glands of baby chicks. Like ACTH, and for routine toxicological assessment of TSH, many tests involve the measurement of target organ secretory responses. The evaluation of TSH often employs the measurement of thyroxine (T_4) and triiodothyronine (T_3).

Several chemicals, environmental factors and pathological states can affect thyroid hormone secretion (Thomas and Bell, 1982; Thomas *et al.,* 1989). Certain foodstuffs and plants contain chemicals (i.e. goitrogens) that can acts as antithyroidal agents. Most of these conditions seem to directly affect the thyroid gland rather than interfering with TSH secretion.

TSH can be measured by RIA. Such tests are very sensitive and highly specific but the species from which the antisera are obtained can affect the levels being detected. Cross-reactivity of antisera can occur. There are other physiological and non-physiological factors that can affect the measurement of TSH and thyroid hormones.

Somatotrophin (STH) or growth hormone (GH) appears to exert a variety of complex metabolic actions leading to protein anabolism and a stimulation of RNA synthesis. A deficiency in GH leads to a reduction in the incorporation of amino acids into protein. Growth hormone causes a marked stimulation of cartilaginous growth at the epiphytes of long bones. Human recombinant DNA growth hormone has been approved for therapeutic use by the US Food and Drug Administration (FDA).

Many factors can affect the secretion of GH (Thomas and Thomas, 1988). Hypoglycaemia can cause a sudden and dramatic increase in serum GH. Starvation can affect GH levels, and cold stress or surgical trauma can lead to an increase in serum GH. Drugs and chemicals that affect catecholoamine neurotranmission and the autonomic nerve system can influence GH secretion, GH bioassays have utilized body weight gain tests in hypophysectomized female rats. GII has been assayed growth plate. A sensitive RIA for rat growth hormone and for human growth hormone is available. GH can be measured by one of several immunological methods.

Whether GH is assessed using bioassays or by the more accurate and sensitive RIA, or other immunoassays, the experimental design of either acute or chronic toxicity tests must closely monitor the nutritional status of the animals. Many toxic agents can retard dietary intake and, hence, reduce body weights. Experimental designs employing paired-feeding protocol may help the toxicologist in interpreting GH activity.

Thyroid Gland

An understanding of the physiology of the thyroid is important for understanding its endocrine toxicity (Thomas and Bell, 1982; Thomas and Keenan, 1986). The primary products of the thyroid are the hormones T_4 and T_3. The initial step in the synthesis of these thyroid hormones is the uptake of dietary iodide into the follicular cells of the thyroid in response to thyrotropin (TSH). Following cellular uptake, the iodide is oxidized, possibly through a free radical mechanism, and then combined with the tyrosine components of a protein of form either monoiodotyrosyl or diidotyrosyl residues. Two molecules of the letter can combine form T_4 whereas one molecule of each combine to form T_3. Normally, T_4, predominates over T_3 in the thyroid, although the ratio can be altered under certain pathological conditions.

T_4 and T_3 can be incorporated into thyroglobulin, which is stored in the follicular colloid material of the thyroid gland. In response to TSH, T_4 and T_3 release results from their proteolytic cleavage from thyroglobulin. Normally, thyroglobulin does not enter the circulation. Monoiodotyronsine and diiodotyrosine can also be released this stage: however, before reaching the circulation they are enzymatically degraded. The liberated iodine in the form of iodide is eventually reincorporated into protein by the thyroid gland.

T_3 and T_4 are transported in the plasma in association with proteins. Although there are species differences in the protein-binding patterns of the thyroid hormones, the primarily binding protein in humans is called thyroxine-binding globulin (TBG). It is an acidic glycoprotein with a molecular weight of 40,000 daltons. It binds T_4 with a relatively high binding affinity and T_3 with a lower affinity. A second transport protein called thyroxine-binding pre-albumin, although present in higher amounts than thyroxine-binding globulin, has a lower binding affinity for the thyroid hormones and is considered of secondary importance. In humans, and most other mammals, the thyroid hormones can secondarily bind to albumin,.

As a consequence of thyroid plasma protein binding, less than 0.1 per cent of the total plasma thyroid hormones exist in a free or unbound form. Care must be exercised when monitoring thyroid function is a species like the rat which does not possess a TBG (i.e. high affinity binding protein). Therefore, the rat has lower plasma levels of protein-bound thyroid hormone. Also, because it is the free form of the hormone which is available for degradation, it is not unreasonable to expect that the plasma half-life for T_4 would be longer in a species with a TBG than in a species without one. The T_4 plasma half-life in the human, which has a TBG, is 5-9 days; in the rat, which does not have a TBG, the T_4 plasma half-life is only 12-24 h.

There are several biochemical steps in the biosynthesis of T_3 and T_4 where toxic chemicals can interfere with thyroid function. They can be categorized by their mechanism of toxic action(s). Stress is a common factor in conditions leading to reduced T_3 syndromes both in animals and humans. The stress may be either thermal or non-thermal. Cold is well known for its actions in stimulating thyroid gland activity. Decreased serum T_3 in starved rats is primarily the result of diminished thyroid secretion of T_4. Experience with laboratory rats has also revealed that a variety of physical and environmental factors also can alter circulating (i.e. plasma) levels of TBG, T_4 and/or T_3.

Many drugs possess side-effects that can interfere with thyroid gland function. Salicylates, anticoagulants phenytoin an other classes of drugs can reduce thyroid function. Propylthiouracil (PTU), a therapeutic drug use in the treatment of hyperthyroidism, decrease T_3 and T_4. PTU is but one drug in a large chemical class of thyroid inhibitors. Phenoxyisobutyrate derivatives, such as clofibrate, induce morphological changes in the thyroid gland.

Diproteverin, a calcium channel blocking agent with anti-anginal properties, causes hypertrophy of thyroid follicular epithelium. Its actions appear to result from enhanced binding and clearance of unconjugated T_4 with a subsequent increase in serum TSH. Amiodarone, and antiarrhythmic drug, often causes thyroid disorders (Rani, 1990). It is an iodine-rich agent which can cause either hypo- or hyperthyrodism after prolonged therapy. Amiodarone has specific inhibitory effects on against-stimulated functions in thyroid cells, probably by interfering with TSH-receptor interactions.

A large number of chemical agents influence the binding, distribution and metabolism of thyroid alterations in thyroid function, primarily because of endocrine regulatory mechanisms. Long-term thyroid hormone derangement caused by xenobiotics may lead to follicular cell carcinogenesis (Hill *et al.*, 1989). It is difficult to use the rodent model for studying the effects in humans because rodents lack TBG. TBG serves as an important buffer system in the control of thyroid hormones. Toxicology studies have to consider that chemicals or drugs frequently act at different levels of thyroid hormone synthesis, utilization and excretion. This action is particularly evident when there is a structural relationship between T_3 or T_4 and the chemical or drug (e.g. phenytoin-DPH).

There are both natural and synthetic agents that can affect the thyroid glands (Donaldson, 1980; Thomas and Keenan, 1986). There are several plant toxins that are consideral natural goitrogens. Vegetables of the cabbage family such as broccoli, brussels sprouts, cauliflower, horse-radish, mustard seed and turnips contain a chemical class of compounds known as glucosinolates. Glucosinolates can be biotransformed into thiocyanates and isothiocyanates which are potent natural goitrogens. Likewise, onions, garlic and chives contain 5-substituted cysteine sulphoxides which are also natural goitrogens. Raw soyabeans, especially if there is inadequate iodine uptake, may produce simple goitres. Heating or cooking the soybeans destroys the natural goitrogens. Cassava a starchy plant, contains considerable amounts of hydrogen cyanide that can cause an increased incidence of goitres.

A number of synthetic herbicides can produce alternations in thyroid gland activity (Stevens and Summer, 1991). There are also a number of chemical classes of herbicides, including chloringated phenylureas, substituted uracils, pyridazinones and diphenyl others. Nitrofen, a halogenated nitrophenol that is selective pre-and postemergence herbicide, reduces follicular size and colloidal density. Triazines are an important class of herbicides that suppress thyroid activity. In animals, long-term feeding studies with amitrole produce thyroid adenonmas and adenocarcinomas. Amitrole inhibits thyroid peroxidase, leading to an increased TSH and goitrogenicity (Rani, 1990). Aminothiazole exerts a direct action on the thyroid by inhibiting. T_4 synthesis and also accelerates its deiodination. 2,4-D can decrease serum protein-bound iodine. Fungicides (e.g. nabam, zineb and zuram) are capable of inhibiting iodine uptake by the thyroid. Chlorine dioxide, sometimes used as an alternative disinfectant in municipal water supplies, reportedly decreases T_4 levels in primates.

It is obvious that many chemicals and drugs can alter thyroid function. The mechanism of toxicological action varies, ranging from inhibiting the anion pump in the thyroid to reducing T_3 and T_4 synthesis.

Adrenal Glands

The adrenal gland has distinct anatomical zones that exert different hormonal and neural actions. The adrenal medulla secretes adrenaline (epinephrine) and noradrenaline (norepinephrine) in response to sympathetic nerve stimulation, and their release produces systemic effects resembling generalized sympathetic stimulation. The adrenal cortex produces who principal groups of steroid hormones, the mineralocorticoids and the glucocorticoids, although small amounts of androgenic hormones may also be secreted.

The primary mineralocorticoid in humans is aldosterone although deoxycorticosterone also exhibits mineralocorticoid activity. Cortisol, the major glucocorticoid produced in humans, also exhibits a low level of mineralocorticoid activity. The physiological action of aldosterone is to modulate electrolyte levels. It promotes the renal reabsorption of sodium in the ascending portion of the loop of Henle, the distal tubule, and in the collecting tubule. The reabsorption of sodium is also accompanied by the reabsorption of chloride anion. In addition to stimulating the reabsorption of sodium aldosternone also enhances the urinary excretion of potassium and hydrogen ions. The increased elimination of hydrogen ions can lead to alkalosis and an increased extracellular content of bicarbonate ions, which when combined with increased extracellular sodium and chloride content, rend to promote the tubular reabsorption of water.

The adrenal cortex is necessary for survival. Without mineralocorticoids, the extracellular fluid potassium concentration rises, and the sodium and chloride content falls. Total lack of aldosterone secretion causes the urinary elimination of 20 per cent of the total body sodium in 1 day. The sodium elimination can cause a dangerous reduction in the extracellular and blood volume which, if not restored, will lead to diminished cardiac output and death.

The glucocorticoids secreted in humans are cortisol or hydrocortisone, although both corticosterone and cortisone possess some glucocorticoid activity. Glucocorticoids regulate carbohydrate, protein and fat metabolism. With carbohydrate metabolism, the glucocorticoids stimulate gluconeogenisis and decrease glucose utilization. Both these effects can lead to increased blood glucose levels. Glucocorticoids produce a marked reduction in cellular protein content, although hepatic protein increases, as does the production of plasma protein by the liver. It is believed that glucocorticoids interfere with the transport of amino acids it extrahepatic cells, and combined with continuing protein catabolism in these cells results in an increase in plasma amino acids. Increased plasma amino acids levels and their subsequent transport into the liver probably promotes gluconeogensis. The gluycocorticoids also promote the mobilization of fatty acids from adipose tissue which elevates plasma fatty acid levels. This effect, plus an increased oxidation of fatty acids in the cells, is probably involved in the switch from glucose utilization to fatty acid utilization as a source of energy during periods of stress.

Corticosteroids are bound to plasma proteins. Corticosteroid-binding globulin (CBG) has a high affinity, but a low binding capacity. Conversely, plasma albumin has a low affinity and a relatively high binding capacity. Physiologically, most of the hormone will be bound to CBG, pharmacological doses quickly overload the total binding site on CBG. Several agents can adversely affect adrenocortical function (Thomas and Keenan 1986; Colby, 1988). If a compound does not produce detectable morphological damage to the adrenal following repeated administration, it is usually accepted that no adrenotoxicity has occurred. This is not to assume that toxicity will pass undetected, particularly considering the influence that adrenocortial hormones have no plasma electrolytes, and carbohydrate, protein and fat metabolism. The guinea-pig is a particularly useful model to study the actions of chemicals or drugs on the adrenal gland. The guinea-pig has, perhaps, the largest adrenal gland/body weight ratio of any animal model. Besides its large size, it is readily dissected into functional zones. Like humans, the guinea-pig has adrenal glands that are very adept at metabolizing xenobiotics (Colby, 1988).

Among the endocrine target organs, the adrenal cortex seems to be particularly susceptible to chemical insult. A host of agents have been reported to produce morphological or functional lesions in the gland. These lesions may be highly localized and in specific anatomical areas of the adrenal cortex. Chemical-induced functional deficits can produce physiological deficits. Carbon tetrachloride produces adrenocortical necrosis, but its locus of toxicity is only the innermost region of the gland, i.e. the zona reticularis. On the other hand, spironolactone, a mineralocorticoid antagonist, produces functional lesions in the zona fasciculata of the adrenal cortex. DDT metabolites (e.g. 3-methylsulphonyl-DDE) (Jonsson *et al.*, 1999) exert their adrenotoxicity by specifically binding to a non-extractable residue in the zona fassiculata. Thus, particular agents have a propensity to affect certain subpopulations of cells within the adrenal cortex. While the adrenal medulla can be adversely affected by various chemicals, by far the majority of chemicals lesions are associated with the adrenal cortex.

Chemicals or drugs that affect the brain or adenhypophysis leading to changes in ACTH secretion will, or course, alter the secretory rate of adrenal steroids Likwise agents affecting the renin-angiotensin system can affect mineralocorticoid secretion. Chemicals can either directly or indirectly affect adrenal cortical function. The response of the adrenal gland to ACTH may be compromised by chemically induced changes on membrane receptors, cyclic nucleotide levels, protein synthesis and other biochemical processes involved in stimulating steroidogenesis. Thus change in biochemical processes in adrenal cortical secretion caused by chemicals can be mediated by several different mechanisms. The adrenal cortex is vulnerable to many different chemicals and through different process. The vascularity of adrenal cortex is excellent so that the delivery of toxic agents is seldom a limiting factor. It is rich in lipids and, hence, fatsoluble toxins are readily assimilated and sequestered in the adrenal gland. The capacity of the adrenal cortex to metabolize foreign substances is, in part, a result of its high concentration of cytochrome P-450. Hence, xenobiotics can undergo detoxification. Alternatively, the metabolism of a xenobiotic may also lead to more toxic intermediates. Bioactivation, or producing more active metabolites, may actually be associated with intermediates with greater inherent toxicities. Toxic metabolities tend to be highly reactive with their concentration usually reaching high local levels producing chemical lesions.

The mechanism of toxic action of spironolactone on the adrenal cortex has been studied extensively (Colby, 1988). Spironolactone is a modified steroid that is a mineralocortiocid antagonist. It competes for aldosterone receptors in the kidney and thus us is used as a diuretic. Spironolactone has both renal and extrarenal site of acting. Its extrarenal sites of action include the liver, the adrenal cortex and the tests. In the tests, spironolactone is more potent in inhibiting steroidogenesis when compared with several other drugs. Aminoglutethimide, a potentadrenolytic agent, can also inhibit gonadal steroidogenesis. The chemicals or drugs that inhibit adrenal gland steroidogenesis can often inhibit testicular steroidogenesis (Thomas and Keenan, 1986; Brun *et al.,* 1991).

The pancreas has a role in digestion, and secretes two importnat hormones, insulin and glucagon. These hormones are synthesized in the islets of Langerhans by *beta* cells (insulin) and *alpha* cells (glucagon). A primary concern, when testing for toxicity of an experimental drug, is the potential for the compound to interfere with the normal functioning of the pancreatic *beta* cells. Often, pancreatic toxicity is heralded by hyperglycaemia and although increased blood glucose might be found during routine clinical chemistry, additional tests are required to pinpoint specific toxicity.

The relationship between insulin and carbohydrate, fat and protein metabolism, can be appreciated by studying diabetes mellitus. In diabetes mellitus, hyperglycaemia results from an impaired utilization of glucose. The failure of glucose to penetrate adipose tissue will mobilize fat, producing a rise in the free fatty acid and triglycride content of plasma and the triglyceride content of the liver. A fatty liver in the diabetic may occur from the absence of lipoprotein synthesis owing to accelerated gluconeogenesis. When glucose oxidation is impaired, fatty acids form the major source of energy; however, this generates an excess of intermediary metabolits, collectively described as ketone bodies (acetone, acetoacetic acid, and β-hydroxybutyric acid), which can lead to the development of metabolic acidosis.

Hyperglycaemia also can lead to the appearance of glucose in the urine (glycosuria) when the blood glucose levels exceed the renal threshold of approximately 180 mg dl^{-1} of blood. At lower blood glucose levels, all the filtered ketose is normally reabsorbed by the renal tubules. Increased blood levels of glucose leading of glycosuria can be caused by emotional stress and the concomitant release of glucose from liver glycogen in response to adrenaline. Glycosuria also can be the consequence of impaired renal tubular function caused by compounds such as the glycoside, or phlorizing. Renal glycosuria, irrespective of the underlying cause, can produce an osmotic diuretic effect which can lead to dehydration and polydipsia. Glycogenolysis and gluconeogensis are increased in diabetes, generating glucose which further enhances hyperglycaemia.

Diabetes mellitus is not a single disease entity. Rather, it represents a heterogeneous groups of glucose intolerance pathologeies evidenced by expression of fasting hyperglycaemia. It may or may not be caused by an absolute or relative deficiency of insulin. Thus, NIDDM and IDDM appear to be separate diseases with different aetiologties. IDDM often involves a development of autoimmunity against β-cells. NIDDM involves genes that are associated with obesity and/or insulin resistance and not with genes that affect the immune system.

Several chemicals or drugs can actually be toxic to pancreatic β cells. From a structural view, there are virtually no chemical similarities among these various agents. This suggests different mechanisms of toxic action(s). Alloxan has been used for many years to purposely destroy pancreatic β cells in an effort to produce experimental diabetes. It has an avidity for β cells and concentrates in this target organ. Alloxan destroyed β cell function leading to hyperglycaemia and glycosuria in experimental animals. Alloxan is rapidly biometabolized to dialuric acid, a product that undergoes autoxidation to yield amounts of peroxide, superoxide anion and free radicals. On the other hand, the toxic action(s) of streptozotocin may reside in the fact that it contains an *N*-methynitrosourea moiety. Streptozotocin is also an alkylating agent. Both alloxan and steptozotocin produce damage to pancreatic DNA.

Diabetogenic agents are effective in producing hyperglycaemia in several species including humans. The pharmacological and toxicological spectrum may differ but their common adverse action resides in their ability to cause varying degrees of destruction of pancreatic β cells. Although alloxan was probably the first agent used to cause β cell necrosis, it has largely been replaced by the methylnitrosourea analogue, streptozotocin, to produce experimental insulin-dependent diabetes. Cyprophetadine, pentamidine and hexamethylmelamine are also capable of suppressing the function and altering the morphology of insulin-secreting cells. Other drugs, such as phenytoin (DPH) and diaoxide (proglycem) can exert an hibitory effect on insulin secretion. They may also act by preventing the peripheral utilization of glucose. Conversely, oral hypoglycaemic drugs (e.g. sulphonylures) can stimulate β cell secretion and are used therapeutically in NIDDM (type II). Cyclosporin, a potent immunosuppressant agent, reduces the requirement for insulin in IDDM (Type I), but its mechanism of action on the β cell remains largely unknown. Finally, cholecystokinin, an endogenous hormone that can physiologically enhance insulin secretion, can be antagonized by experimental agents such as loxiglumide (Hildebrand *et al.,* 1991).

Not only are β cells destroyed by rather specific chemicals, but some species (or strains) are more or less susceptible to genetically induced diabetes mellitus. Thus, experimental animals models for diabetes mellitus may exploit genetic susceptibility or may involve chemically induced destruction of β cells. A number of inbred strains of mice are sensitive to *db* gene-induced diabetes with sexual dimorphism in some inbred strains emphasizing the relationship between the obesity gene and sex. The major genetic regulator to inbred strain diabetogenic sensitivity is sex-related. In the rat, the BHE strains is an excellent animal model for the study of NIDDM (Berdanier, 1991).

Considerable progress has also been made in culturing pancreatic islet cells, hence affording an important *in vitro* model to study insulin secretion. Insulinoma cell lines have contributed greatly to studies of morphology and function of islet cells, which are relevant to the aetiology of diabetes mellitus. Progress in tissue culture for the transplantation of islets cells across major histocopatibility barriers may lead to replacement therapy for diabetic patients. Artificial pancreas implants in experimental animals may eventually advance to where the concept can be used in diabetic patients requiring islet cell replacement. Recently, a hybrid pancreas consisting of a plastic housing containing a coiled membrance surrounded by living pancreas cells has been shown to be effective in secreting insulin and modulating blood glucose levels.

It is also possible to destroy the α cells of the pancreas somewhat selectively. There are species differences with regard to α cell destruction. The injection of cobalt chloride has been shown to produce degranulation and vacuolization of the α cells in rabbits, dogs and guinea pigs. Synthalin A can also selectively cause necrosis of pancreatic α cells.

While attention focuses on those agents that produce destruction of β cells leading to diabetogenic states, there are still many other agents that cause pancratitis (Banerjee *et al.,* 1989; Steer, 1989). Thus, both endocrine and exocrine function of the pancreas are vulnerable to chemical insult. Drugs and chemicals cause acute pancreastitis, but seldom cause chronic pancratitis. Acute pancreatitis is often accompanied by increased blood levels of pancreatic enzymes, notably analyse. The exact mechanism in cellular inflammation is not understood, but several factors may be involved. Pancreatic duty hypertension may lead to autodigestion and necrosis induced inflammation of the pancreas. In animals, choline deficiency coupled with the infusion of caevalin (a pancreozymin-cholecystokinin analogue) leads to acute pancreatitis.

Diuretic-induced changes in electrolytes appear to be correlated with acute pancreatitis, particularly in association with hyperamy-lasaemia. Tetracyclines may exert a direct pancreotoxicity; azahioprine suppresses the immune system yet has a direct cytotoxic action. Other drugs may also possess a direct cyto-toxic action, e.g. valproic acid and possibly L-asparaginase. Alletgic reactions are associated with sulphonamides and their pancreotoxicity. It is evident that many drugs can cause acute pancreatitis but the underlying mechanisms are poorly understood.

9

Poisons of Animal Origin

Poisons of animal organ encompass a broad array of toxic agents that are possessed by thousands of animal species. The vast number of poisonous and venomous animals, as well as significant differences among these species, prohibits generalizations that would be necessary to review this topic extensively. The toxicity of these agents, therefore, will be reviewed by discussing representative animal species that are significant hazards to humans.

It is important first to distinguish between animals that are poisonous and those that are venomous. A venomous animal can produce venom in specialized glands or cells which can be administered in some way to its enemy or prey. Poisonous animals, on the other hand, possess a toxin(S) within their tissue that can have deleterious effects when ingested.

Considerable differences exist within the animal kingdom with respect to the venom apparatus, mode of envenomation and constituents of the venom. Venomous animals can either bite or sting their victims and some are capable of squirting or spitting venom. The venom of most species is a unique but complex proteinaceous mixture. The biochemical and pharmacological properties of most venoms are incompletely understood because of their complexity. Difficulties in obtaining sufficient venom and in extracting individual components further complicate this issue.

An animal may use its venom offensively or defensively. For example it may be used to subdue or kill its prey and to aid in digestion. Alternatively, it may be used to ward off predators. Many venoms are multipurpose and cannot be narrowly classified. The toxic manifestations from envenomation will be influenced by these functiones the corresponding venom constituents.

Most poisonous animals accumulate toxin through the marine food chain. Unicellular sea algae (dinoflagellates) are the most common initial source. A number of these dinoflagellates are responsible for the often publicized 'red tides' which are associated with poisonous shellfish.

Although people who live in regions inhabited by venomous or poisonous animal are at greatest risk for toxic exposure, such encounters can occur elsewhere. Venomous animals, for example, may be imported by hobbyists or shipped inadvertently in produce or other goods. Likewise, poisonous seafood may be shipped to distant markets. This may present a therapeutic dilemma to a practitioner unfamiliar with such exposures. Regional Poison Control Centers are staffed with specially trained professionals who can provide expert information and advice on the management of such cases. These centers also have access to the Antivenom Index which was developed to assist with locating the appropriate antivenin to exotic bites and stings. The Index is a joint effort of the American Association of Zoological Parks and Aquriums, the American Association of Poison Control Centers and the Arizona Poison and Drug Information Center and similar information sources are available in some other countries.

Snakes

Snakes are probably the most well recognized of all venomous animals. Their notorious reputation is established inancient history, myth, magic and religion. While some people adore and are fascinated by these creatures, others are inordinately fearful. As expected, snakes and snakebite have been extensively studied but because of the vast number and complexity of these species and their venoms, considerable work is still needed.

It is estimated that up to 1 million snakebites occur annually worldwide resulting in up to 40,000 deaths. Approximately 45,000 snakebites occur in the USA each year of which 8000 are inflicted by venomous species (Russell *et al.,* 1975). In the USA only about 9-14 deaths occur annually from venomous snakebite (Russell, 1980). In some countries, e.g. the UK, poisonous snakebites are uncommon but venomous snakebite is a much more significant problem in other parts of the world. In India, for example, available data suggests that up to 200,000 snakebites occur annually with approximately 15,000 deaths (George *et al.,* 1987). Most bites are inflicted on the foot or leg. Accidental snakebites occur most often in children during daylight hours of warm summer months. Conversely, adult men are frequently victims of snakebites that could be easily avoided, bites which have been termed illegitimate.

Over 3000 species of snakes are distributed throughout the world, primarily in temperate climates. Approximately 300 of these snakes are significantly hazardous to humans. Snakes are members of the class Reptilia. There are five families of venomous snakes including the Colubridae, Crotalidae, Elapidaee, Hydophidae and Viperidae.

Only two snakes in the family Colubridae are significant hazards to humans, namely the boomslang (*Dispholidus typus*) and vine snake (*Thelotornis capensis*), which are found in southern Africa (Aitchison, 1990). Their venomous bite results primarily in a consumptive coagulopathy, delayed haemorrage and related complications. Crotalidae species are distributed throughout the world and include the pit vipers such as rattlesnakes, copper heads and cottonmouths. These snakes most notably produce local tissue necrosis and coagulopathies. Elapids, which are found in Asia. Australia, Africa and the Americas, include such notorious creatures as cobras, mambas and coral snakes (Russell, 1983; Nelson, 1989). Predominantly neurotoxic effects result from the venomous bites of these snakes. The Viperidae family includes the vipers, located in Africa, Europe and Middle East (Nelson, 1989). The toxic effects of their bites are comparable to those of the Crotalidae. The Hydrophids include the sea snakes which are found in warm, shallow waters in the Indian and Pacific Oceans (Tu and Fulde, 1987). Although these snakes possess very potent neurotoxins, their short fangs and low venom output results in relatively few serious envenomations.

Toxic Manifestations

Snakes are often categorized by the primary toxic effects of their venom but this oversimplifies the problem. For example, several species of cobra, whose venoms are considered neurotoxic, may also produce significant local necrosis as well as potentially lethal cardiotoxic events (Blaylock, 1982; Kunkel *et al.,* 1983-84; Minton, 1990). Likewise, rattlesnakes generally produce local tissue damage and coagulopathies but minimal neurotoxicity. The bite of the Mojave rattlesnake (*Crotalus scutulatus*), however, produces less local swelling and pain but neurotoxicity can be a significant problem (Russell *et al.,* 1975; Kunkel *et al.,* 1983-84).

Snake venom is as complex mixture of protein, enzymes, metals and other inorganic substances (Russell, 1983). The venom of some species, in fact, may contain you to 20 different components (Russell, 1983). However, relatively little is known about the composition of most venoms. The complex nature of snake venom as well as intra-and interspecies differences contribute to the variability and perplexity of snake venom poisoning.

The potential severity of envenomation is dependent on a number of factors, including the species of snake involved; its age and size; the location, number and depth of bites; and the total quantity of venom injected. Other important factors include the age and size of the victim and their general state of health. Not all strikes by snakes result in envenomation. So called 'dry bites' may occur in up to 30 per cent of crotalid bites, 50 per cent of elapid bites, and up to 75 per cent of sea snake bites.

Local Toxic Effects

Envenomation by Crotalids and Viperids typically results in significant local toxic effects. Pain, swelling and oedema occur soon after the bite. In severe cases the oedema progresses rapidly. Within several hours the site may become ecchymotic and discoloured. Vesicles may also appear, which are usually filed with clear fluid become filled with blood in severe cases. Local tissue necrosis may also occur which is probably due to the direct action of the venom's enzymes. Pain and swelling are generally most severe following bites by eastern and western diamond back rattlesnakes and least severe following bites by copperheads and *Sistrurus* rattlesnake species.

Coagulopathies

Snake envenomation may result in a variety of systemic manifestations. Probably the most significant but unpredictable are coagulopathes. Snakes within all families have been implicated with such disorders. Both anticoagulant and procoagulant properties have been described but bleeding disorders occur most commonly.

Anticoagulation results from the constituents of snake venom that may (1) interfere with activation of clotting factors, (2) have fibrionlytic and fibrinogenolytic activity, (3) directly or indirectly activate plasminogen, or (4) directly act on phospholipids (Russell, 1983). Thrombocytopenia with or without other coagulopathies may result from intravascular clotting and consumption of platelets, sequestration of platelets at the site of envenomation or destruction of platelets by the venom (Riffer *et al.,* 1987). The degree of thrombocytopenia may directly correlate with the severeity of envenomation (La Grange and Russell, 1970). Disseminated intravascular coagulation may complicate severe cases.

Snake venom constituents may interact at various

points of the coagulation cascade to activate clotting factors or been prothrombin directly (Russell, 1983). Significant amounts of thrombin like enzymes have also been identified in the venom of crotalids and viperids (Russell, 1983).

Cardiotoxicity

Cardivascular shock is a common cause of death from crotalid envenomation and contributed to other systemic complications (Hardy, 1986). Shock results from increased capillary permeability which leads to third-spacing of fluids and intravascular volume depletion (Schaeffer *et al.*, 1979). Reduced cardic output secondary to venon-induced cardiac changes, as well as the release of mediators such as bradykinins, histamine and serotonin, may also contribute to haemodynamic compromise.

Neurotoxicity

Neurotoxicity is primarily associated with enveomation by elapids and hydrophids. The venoms of these snakes are comparable but the venoms of sea snakes are more toxic. The neurotoxin of sea snakes binds to postsynaptic acetylcholine receptors resulting in paralysis. Respiratory paralysis is the primary cause of immediate death (Kitchens and van Mierop, 1987). The venom of elapids such as the banded krait contains presynaptic neurotoxins which inhibits the release of acetylcholine at the myoneural junction. Neurotoxic signs and symptoms include diplopia, slurred speech, deafness paraesthesias, hyperaesthesia, muscle fasciculations, weakness, incoordination, trisums, pain, stiffness, drowsiness, apprehension, increased salivation, diaphoresis and convulsions. Crotalid envenomation can also cause perioral paraesthesiasm muscle fasciculations and weakness. The Mojave rattlesnake (*Crotalus scutulatus*) is a unique crotalid in that neurotoxic manifestations predominate.

Other Toxic Manifestations

Numerous other systemic toxic effects have been

associated with snake bites. These may result from either direct actions of the venom or as complications of cardiovascular, neuromuscular or coagulation disorders. Renal failure may complicate crotalidae, hydrophidae and viperidae enrvenomation, which may result from disseminated intravascular coagulation, cardiovascular shock or hemolysis. A direct nephrotoxic effect of the venom is postulate as the primary cause of renal failure in *Vepera russelli* envenomation. Adult respiratory distress syndrome may developing severe cases. The aretiology is unclear but shock, disseminated intravascular coagulation, multiple blood component transfusions and the venom itself are all postulated.

Management

A shroud of controversy veils the treatment of venomous snakebite. Rather than fully exploring all treatment issues and modalities, an overview of the generally accepted approach to management will be presented.

The most important first aid measures are to keep the victim calm, immobilize the bitten extremity and transport to the nearest appropriate health care facility. Incision and suction to the bite is generally impractical and potentially dangerous. It may be beneficial in a few select cases when it can be performed within a few minutes by a qualified individual using appropriate equipment. Likewise, the use of a lymphatic tourniquet to impede venom distribution is of questionable value and hazardous if done improperly. The use of a firm bandage wrapped around the affected extremity in conjunction with immobilization has been shown to delay elapid venom distribution (Sutherland *et al.*, 1979). Such an approach may have some utility in the management of elapid or hydrophid bites. The bandage is contraindicated following bites by snakes that cause necrosis such as the crotalids and viperids. Cryotherrapyis also ciontraindicated.

Correct identification of the offending snake is important. Unfortunately, the victim often cannot give a detailed description of the snake and it is usually not available for examination. The use of immunological tests to identify snake venom is serum or other materials is currently used in some parts of the world. In Australia, for example, venom detection kits, which use the enzyme-linked immunosorbent assay (ELISA) technique, are an integral part of snakebite management.

Antivenin therapy is the cornerstone of snakebite management worldwide. The choice of antivenin depends on the species of snake involved and available forms of antivenin. Antivenin may be monovalent (activity against only one species of snake) or polyvalent (activity against two or more species of snake). If available, monovalent antivenin is preferable when the offending species of snake is known with certainty. Polyvalent anti-venins have been developed to treat many venomous species in geographical area. In the USA, for example, Antivenin (Crotalidae) Polyvalent (Wyeth Laboratories, Philadelphia, PA) is active against all pit vipers in the western hemisphere and even some Asian species.

The clinical status of the patient and the species of snake involved guide antivenin therapy. It first must be determined if the patient was envenomated. The patient should be closely monitored for the development of local or systemic signs or symptoms as well as laboratory changes. Approximately 4-6 h of observation is generally necessary to rule out significant envenomation. There are, however, notable exception to these fundamental guidelines. Bites by the eastern coral snake (*Micrurus fulvius*), for example, may produce minimal local toxic effects, but profound neurotoxicity may develop hours later, Likewise, the Mojave rattlesnake (*Crotalus scutulatus*) may produce minimal local effects, but neurotoxic manifestations can be delayed. Accordingly, prophylactic antivenin therapy is indicated for all definite bites by the eastern coral snake and other potentially neurotoxic envenomations.

The dose of antivenin is dependent on the species of the snake, the particular antivenin, and the severity of the envenomation. If indicated, antivenin should be administered as soon as possible following the bite. It is important to note that children should receive the same dose of antivenin as would an adult and possibly even more.

The initial dose of Antivenin (Crotalidae) Polyvalent for crotalid bites depends on the initial severity of the bite. Russell recommends grading the severity as minimal, moderate or severe (Russell, 1983). Minimal envenomations involve only local manifestations confined to the area of the bite and should be treated with three to five vials of antivenin. Moderate envenomations that involve progressive local effects, significant systemic manifestations and laboratory changes should be treated with six to ten vials. Severe envenomation, which should be treated initially with at least ten vials of antivenin, involves the entire extremity or part and there is serious systemic toxicity and laboratory changes. Additional doses of antivenin may needed if toxic effects persist following the initial dose (Russell, 1980). In severe cases 30 or more vials may be required.

All currently available snake antivenin are derived from hyperimmunized horse serum. As a result some patients will develop an immediate type I hypersensitivity reaction, which is IgE mediated (Otten and McKimm, 1983). To reduce the risk of unexpected hypersensitivity reactions all patients should be skin tested prior to administering any antivenin. In the event of an allergic response the potential risks and benefits from therapy must be weighed. Generally, if life or limb is at stake, antivenin therapy should be continued after taking appropriate precautions. Patients who are treated with antivenin also are likely to develop a delayed immune complex reaction commonly known as serum sickness. This is an IgG-and IgM-medicated process which results in the formation of antigen-antibody complexes and the subsequent activation of the complement system. Acute IgE-mediated allergic reactions to antigens in the snake venom itself have also been reported.

The allergenic nature of currently available antivenin is a significant limitation. It causes indecision as to whether to start therapy and restricts the dose of antivenin that can be safely administered. This is compound by the fact that in some cases many vials of currently available antivenins are needed to adequately neutralize the venom. A promising approach to resolve this dilemma is the use of polyacrylamide gel affinity chromatography to produce purified antibodies (Russell *et al.,* 1985). The superior efficacy and safety of this product has been demonstrated in both *in vivo* and *in vitro* studies (Russell *et al.,* 1985). Purified Fab fragments of IgG may provide further pharmacokinetic, therapeutic and safety advantages. The application of monoclonal antibody technology may be useful for those species whose venom contains one main toxin, such as the elapids. The use of monoclonal antibodies for crotalids or viperids, on the other hand, is impractical because of the complexity of their venoms.

Local wound care should be provided as needed and tetanus immunization should be updated if necessary. The systemic manifestations of poisonous snakebite are managed with traditional supportive measures. As intravascular volume depletion is a primary cause of cardiovascular shock, adequate fluid replenishment is essential. Central venous pressure (CVP) and pulmonary artery wedge pressure (PAWP) should be used to guide therapy. Oxygen should be administered and appropriate respiratory support provided as needed. Whole blood or blood products may be needed to treat acute blood loss and coagulopathies. The use of anticholinesterase agents such as neostigmine bromide has been suggested as a means to treat the paralysis of elapid bites (Blaylock, 1982). Antivenin and appropriate supportive measures, however, should be sufficient.

Gila Monster

The Gila Monster, *Heloderma suspectum,* is one of a few known venomous lizards. There are five subspecies of Heloderma including: *Heloderma suspectum suspectum* and *H. s. cintum* (banded Gila monster), which are found in south-western USA; *H. horridum horridum* (beaded lizard)

H. h, exasperatum and *H. h. alvarez,* which along with *H. s. suspectum* are found in Mexico (Russell and Boget, 1981). *H. h. alvarez* and *H. h. horridum* are also located further south into Guatemala.

The Gila monster may be kept as an exotic pet; therefore, humans may be bitten and require treatment essentially anywhere. In fact, most bites by venomous lizard result from careless handling rather than unsuspecting attacks in nature.

The Gila monster is a rather large, slow moving, nocturnal reptile. Adults may reach 55 cm in length (Russell and Boget, 1981). They feed mostly on small animals and have few predators others than humans.

The Helodermatids have a much less sophisticated venom apparatus than snakes. It consists of two venom glands located in the lower law. A pair of venom ducts lead to venom-conducting grooved teeth. When the Gila monster bites, it passively injects venom as its drawn up its teeth by capillary action.

The venom apparatus is used primarily in defence. When the Gila monster bites, it often holds on crush its prey and to allow suffi-cient venom to be injected. The venom contains proteins and a number of enzymes. Serotonin, amine oxidase, phospholipase A, protease, lipase and hyaluronidase have all been identified. The venom may also have bradykinin-releasing activity.

Toxic Manifestations

There have been sporadic reports of humans bitten by the Gila monster. The bite generally results in relatively minor local and systemic toxic effects. On the other hand, life-threatening reactions have been reported. Bites should be treated, therefore, as medical emergencies with appropriate evaluation and care.

The Gila monster has strong jaws which can inflict significant local pain from mechanical trauma. Several small puncture wounds may results. Occasionally teeth may become lodged in the tissue. Bluish discoloration around the bite may be noted but tissues necrosis is unlikely. Injected venom caused pain which can be intense and may radiate throughout the extremity.

Oedeman generally develops more slowly and is less severe than that which occurs with snake bites but in some cases it can become quite marked and tense (Roller, 1976; Russell and Bogert, 1981). This may contribute to the pain of ennomation. Lymphadenopathy and lymphadenitis have also been reported (Russell and Bogert, 1981; Bou-Abboud and Kardasskis, 1988).

Other common manifestations include weakness, faintness or dizziness, diaphoresis, nausea, vomiting and hypotension. Profound hypotension has been reported in several cases (Heitschel, 1986; Piacentine *et al.,* 1986; Streiffer, 1986; Bou Abboud and Kardassakis, 1988; Preston,1989).

Other cardiovascular effects have been described including nonspecific electrocardiogram changes, ventricular arrythmias, and myocarial infraction (Roller, 1976; Bou-Abboud and Kardassakis, 1988; Streiffer, 1986; Preston, 1989). Impaired renal function has also been reported which is probably a result of prolonged hypotension (Preston, 1989).

Laboratory abnormalities may include hypokalaemia and leucocytosis. Thrrombocytopenia has been rarely reported. Thrombocytopenia associated with reduced fibrinogen and increased prothrombin time, partial thromboplastin time and fibrin split products indicated a consumptive coagulopathy in two cases (Bou-Abboud and Kardassakis, 1988; Preston, 1989).

Management

Limited first aid can be provided. The first step often is to remove the lizard, which can be difficult. Several reasonable approaches include : (1) using a stick of similar device inserted in the back of the jaw of pry it off; (2) putting the affected extremity under water thereby causing the animal to release itself; or (3) lighting and holding a match under the Gila monster's jaw. Keep the patient warm immobilize the extremity and transport to an appropriate health care facility.

The site of the bite should be thoroughly cleansed and examined for remaining teeth. An X-ray of the site may be helpful.

There is no commercially available Gila monster antivenin. Vital signs and laboratory indices should be monitored closely. An electrocardiogram should also be obtained. Treatment is primarily symptomatic and supportive care.

Hymenoptera

Flying insects of the order hymenoptera are distributed worldwide. A few of the thousands of known species are significantly hazardous to humans. These include honeybees, bumblebees, wasps, hornets and yellow jackets. Honeybee and bumblebees belong to the family Apidae; the others belongs to the family Vespidae.

The vespids are generally more aggressive and attack vigorously if disturbed. Honeybees account for most apidae and a person is most likely to be stung by honeybees when around flowering plants. Yellow jackets tend to nest on the ground or in decaying wood. They will scavenge for food and may be pests at picnics or around garbage cans. Hornets build nests in tress or shrubs; wasps often nest under eaves of buildings.

Their stinging apparatus consists of a modified ovipositor that is connected to a venom sac. They grasp the victim's skin with their claws and then jab their stinger into the skin. The stinger of honeybees is barbed so it and the venom sac remain attached to the victim's skin when the bee flies away resulting in its demise. Vespids and the bumblebee are generally able to withdraw their stingers and are capable of stinging again. Some yellow jackets, however, may also lose their stinger.

Stings from these insects may resulting manifestations ranging from minor local pain and swelling to life-threatening respiratory and cardiovascular compromise. These toxic effects may result from direct local and systemic effects of the venom as well as allergic reactions to venom proteins.

Toxic Manifestations

Up to 50 µl of venom may be injected with each sting. This dose is insufficient to produce systemic toxicity; however, venom constituents will produce local irritation and pain. If a person is stung many times at once then sufficient venom may be injected to produce toxicity. Systemic toxicity from bee stings resembles an allergic reaction. Toxicity from vespid stings may include an acute allergic-like response followed by delayed effects such as haemolysis, habdomyolysis and renal failure (Bousquet *et al.,* 1984).

The normal response to a hymenoptera sting consists of a small painful, urticarial lesions that lasts only a few hours. Approximately 10-17 per cent of people may develop a large local reaction that includes swelling and erythema greater than 5 cm in diameter which may last more than 24 h (Maguire and Geha, 1986; Reisman, 1989). This large local reaction may have an immunological origin.

The allergic reactions to hymenoptera stings deserve detailed discussion. The allergic response may range from exaggerated local effects to analphylaxis and death. It is estimated that hymenoptera stings account for at least 40-50 deaths annually in the USA, more deaths than result from all other venomous animals (Golden, 1989). The systemic allergic response to hymenoptera stings is IgE mediated. Recent evidence also suggests a role for indirect complement activation (Valentine *et al.,* 1990). There is considerable cross activity among the various vespids but cross reactivity between vespid and bee venoms is reality uncommon (Wright and Lockey, 1990).

The incidence of systemic allergic reactions may be as low as 0.4-0.8 per cent in children but as high 4.0 per cent in adults (Settipane *et al.,* 1972; Golden *et al.,* 1982). Up to

10-15 per cent of the population may be sensitized to hymenoptera venom but have not had an allergic response (Golden *et al.,* 1982).

Systemic allergic reactions may range from mild, primarily dermatological manifestations to life-threating anaphylxis. Mild systemic reactions consist of generalized urticaria,; angiooedema, erythema and pruritus (Maguire and Geha, 1986). Gastrointestinal gsymptoms may also be present. Laryngeal oedema, bronchospasm and hypotension may be life-threatening in severe cases (Maguire and Geha, 1986).

These are limited data to characterize which patients may develop some, none, or all of these manifestations. Important factors include the age of the patient, history of prior stings, sensitization as documented by skin test or RAST (radioallergosobrent tests) and previous response to hymenoptera stings. Approximately 75 per cent of the population is not sensitized to hyemnoptera venom and will develop a normal local response, and less than 1 per cent will develop a systemic allergic reaction (Golden, 1989). Those who have previously had normal or large local reactions but have a positive skin test or RAST have a 10-20 per cent risk of developing a systemic reaction (Golden, 1989). Patients with a previous history of a systemic reaction who have a positive skin test or RAST have a 50 per cent chance of developing another systemic reaction (Golden, 1989).

It is commonly thought that patients develop more severe reactions with subsequent stings. While it is true that patients who are stung repeatedly within a relatively short time (weeks to months) are more likely to develop a systemic reaction, most patients develop more mild or similar reactions with subsequent stings. Insect sting allergy, in fact, is a self-limiting disease for most people (Reisman, 1989). In other words, the more time between stings the less likely a person is to have a serious systemic reaction.

The typical allergic response in children is much different from that in adults. Children are more likely to have develop cutaneous hypotension (Golden, 1989). Also, children much less frequently develop recurrent systemic manifestations. In fact, children who have previously had non-life-threating allergic reactions are unlikely subsequently to develop a life-threatening creation (Suhuberth *et al.*, 1983; Valentine *et al.*, 1990)

Management

First aid treatment for hymenoptera stings includes removing the stinger (if it remains) by scraping across the site with a blunt-edged object such as credit card. Do not grab the stinger to pull it out as squeezing the venom sack will inject more venom. The area should be washed well with soap and water. Normal local reactions can be managed by applying ice to reduce swelling oedema and pruritus. An antihistamine such as diphenhydramine may also help relieve pruritus. Large local reactions may be helped by elevating the extremity and administering an analgesic as well as glucocorticoid such as prednisone. The combined use of H_1^- and H_2^- antagonists has been suggested as a means to decrease the severity of late phase cutaneous reactions.

Adrenalineis the drug of choice for systemic sting reactions. Subcutaneous administration is adequate in mild to moderate cases. In the event of hypotension, adrenaline (epinephrine) should be administered intravenously. Intravenous fluids and aggressive cardiopulmonary resuscitation should be provided if adrenaline (epinephrine) therapy alone is not adequate. Oral or intravenous antihistamines should only be used for cutaneous manifestations of hymenoptera allergy.

Patients who may develop systemic reactions should be prescribed an emergence kit that includes adrenaline (epinephrine) for subscutaneous injection. This includes those patients with a previous history of systemic allergic effects and those who have had large local reactions and have a positive skin test or RAST.

Venom immune therapy (VIT) may be useful in selected cases. It is presently indicated for those patients who previously have had life-threatning systemic reactions and have a positive skin test or RAST (Maguire and Geha, 1986). Adults are more likely candidates than children as they are at greater risk for developing a repeat systemic reaction. Immunotherapy, in fact, is unnecessary in most children (Valentine *et al.,* 1990). Other patients with less severe systemic reactions who have positive skin tests or RAST may benefit from VIt but the cost of therapy and other factors such as their age, medical history, occupation, outdoor activities or hobbies must be considered.

Ants

Ants belong to the family Formicidae and comprise the third group of venomous hymenoptera. Thousands of ant species are distributed worldwide, some of which can inflict painful venomous stings. Local or systemic allergic reactions can also occur. Not all venomous ants sting. Some, such as the carpenter and weaver ants of the subfamily Formacinae, bite their prey and then spray venom into the wound. Formic acid, which is a potent cytotoxin, is the primary constituent of their venom.

Fire ants (*Solenopsis spp*) are native to both North and South America. Fire ant envenomation is a significant health in the southern USA (Blum, 1984; Stafford *et al.,* 1989a). In fact, up to 60 per cent of the population in an infested area are stung each year (deShazo *et al.,* 1990). The red imported fire ant (*Solenopsis invicta*) has rapidly spread throughout the southern USA and has overtaken the less aggressive native species (*S. xyloni*), as well as the black imported fire ant (*S. richteri*). The imported fire ants of the USA are so named because they are thought to have been introduced via produce shipped from Brazil to Mobile, Alabama in 1939.

Ants sting to subdue their prey and as a means of defence. The fire ant grasp its victim with its mandibles, then using its head as a pivot it swings its abdominal stinger to inflict multiple stings (Diaz *et al.,* 1989). Unlike other hymenoptera, fire ants sting slowly and may inject venom for seconds to minutes (Stafford *et al.,* 1989b). With each sting the ant injects from 0.04 to 0.11 µl of venom (deShaoz *et al.*, 1990).

The venom of most ants and other hymenoptera consists primarily of protein (Blum, 1984). Imported fire ant venom, on the other hand, is 90-95 per cent piperidine alkaloids and contains only 0.1 per cent protein (Hoffman *et al.*, 1988a). Four proteins have been identified, namely: *Sol i I, Sol i II, Sol i III and Sol i IV* (Hoffman *et al.*, 1988a). All these proteins are significant allergens.

Toxic Manifestations

Toxicity associated with fire ant envenomation is normally limited to the site of the sting. *In vitro* studies indicate that the venom has haemolytid, cytotoxic, bactericidal and insecticidal properties (Adrouny *et al.*, 1959; Rhodes *et al.*, 1977). Multiple stings (approximately 10,000), however, have not resulted in systemic toxicity (Diaz *et al.*, 1989).

The local response to envenomation includes an initial weal and false reaction. Superficial vesicles with clear fluid develop the site of the sting within 4 h. This fluid is lost and replaced within 8-10 h by cloudy fluid which becomes purelent. A pustule develops within 24 h which may be surrounded by a red halo (Car *et al.*, 1957). This lesions is pathognomonic in the USA for fire ant stings (Lockey, 1990).

Large local reactions may also occur, which may be immunologically mediated (Diaz *et al.*, 1989). These reactions are characteristics of 'latephase reactions's that occur secondary to ragweed (deShazo *et al.*, 1984). Systemic allergic reactions characteristic or those caused by other hymenoptera may also occur. The natural history of such responses has not been well studied but is probably comparable to that for other hymenoptera. Anaphylxis may result in up to 1 per cent of stings (deShazo *et al.*, 1990).

The prevalence of asymptomatic sensitized people to fire ant venomis comparable to that which exists for other hymenoptera, approximately 16 per cent (Hoffmann *et al.*, 1988b). Crossreactivity may exist between bee or wasp veno and fire ant venom. *Sol i II* has been identified as the crossreactive protein (Hoffman *et al.,* 1988b).

An important complication of fire ant stings is secondary infection (Parrin *et al.,* 1981). Neurological sequelae including serizures and mononeuropathy have also been reported (Fox *et al.,* 1982). The aetiology of such reactions is not known.

Management

First aid for fire ant envenomation is primarily thorough washing with soap and water. Although a number of therapeutic measures have been evaluated as a means of alter the development of pustules, neither topical nor parenteral therapies had any effect developing legions (Parrin *et al.,* 1981). A cold compress may help relieve some swelling and discomfort. The pustules should be bandaged to prevent excoriation. Large local reactions and systemic allergic reactions should be managed as previously described for other hymenoptera.

As with other hymenoptera the indications for immunotherapy are not clear. The relatively high risk for stings in sensitized people, however, causes many to undergo such therapy (Stafford *et al.,* 1989c). To confound the issue further, only whole body extracts are available for therapy, which contain variable quantities of venom. Some evidence of its effectiveness, however, has been presented (Hylander *et al.,* 1989).

Spiders

Spiders are arthropods of the order arachindae. Most spiders are venomous; in fact, all but two families of spiders have venom glands. Thousands of venomous spiders are distributed worldwide; however, only a few are of significant medical importance. Most notable are spiders of the genus *Latrodectus* and *Loxosceles.*

Black Widow Spider

The true black widow spider (*Latrodectus mactans*) is

found in temperature zones of North America including all of the USA except Alaska. Other *Latrodectus* species are distributed throughout the world (Rauber, 1983-84). The major differences between these species are in their body markings and habitats. *L. mactans* has a characteristics shiny black coloration with a red hourglass-shaped marketing on its abdomen. Generally, these spiders are non-aggressive and bite defensively when threatened or disturbed. They are typically found in undisturbed, protected areas such as storage buildings, wood piles and garbage heaps. Females spiders make irregular funnel shaped webs in which to trap prey and suspend their egg sacs.

Only the females of this species are hazardous to humans. The male is too small to cause significant envenomation. The black widow has claw like hollow fangs which are connected to two venom glands in its cepalothorax. The venom glands have striated musculature which controls the injection of venom. While there are some intespecies differences in venom constituents, the toxic fraction appears to be the same (Rauber, 1983-84).

The venom of the black widow, which is one of the most potent of all animal venoms, is primarily neurotoxic. The venom gland contains just less than 0.2 mg venom (Binder, 1989). The mean lethal doses range from 0.005 to 1.0 mg kg^{-1} in various animal species (Edlich *et al.,* 1985). The venom acts at the neuromuscular synaptic junction causing the release of acetylcholine and noradrenaline (norepinephrin) from presynaptic vesicles (Rauber, 1983-84; Binder, 1989). This results in excessive neuromuscular stimulation and, as expected, other cholinergic and adrenergic signs and symptoms. The venom causes initial local muscle pain which then generalizes to involve primarily large muscle groups (Kobernick, 1984).

Toxic Manifestations

Most bites in humans occur above the waist on the forearm or torso (Moss and Binder, 1987). Bites are more prevalent during the late summer or early autumn, a time at which there are increased numbers of both young and mature spiders (Moss and Binder, 1987). Although the bite itself is often not initially painful and may go unnoticed, pain at the site is the most common early symptom of envenomation (Moss and Binder, 1987). Other common symptoms include abdominal pain and cramping as well as lower extremity pain and weakness. Hypertension, tachycardia, fever, leucocytosis, restlessness, mental status changes, headache, rash, paraesthesiae, albuminuria, ptosis, and periorbital oedema safe also been reported. In severe cases shock, coma, respiratory failure and pulmonary oedema may occur. The mortality rate from black widow envenomation is probably less than 1 per cent (Binder, 1989).

Management

There are no specific first aid measures for black widow envenmation. The bite site should be thoroughly cleansed and tetanus immunization should be updated if necessary. Medical management is primarily directed at relieving muscle spasms and pain. Calcium gluconate, administered intravenously, has been shown to be both safe and effective (Binder, 1989). Centrally acting muscle relaxant such as methocarbamol and diazwpam may also provide relief. Dantrolene sodium, a direct-acting muscle relaxant, has been used successfully and is reported to provide more pronounced and protracted relief (Ryan, 1983-84). Narcotic analgesics and sedatives may also be employed to help relieve pain and restlessness.

An equine-derived antivenin is available but is not used routinely in the USA because of the risks associated with horse serum-based produces. In one of a small number of patients there was no demonstrable difference between those who received antivenin and those who did not in terms of length of hospitalization, ancillary drug use for pain control, or clinical outcome (Moss and Binder, 1987). It is generally recommended that antivenin be reserved for cases of severe envenomation in which standard measures are inadequate. It can also be used in life-threatening situations and in those at high risk for severe morbidity, such as the very young or old, and in those with underlying hypertension, cardiac or cerebrovascular disease. As with any equinederived antivenin the risk for hypersensitivity reactions must be considered and appropriate skin testing and other precautions must be taken.

Necrotic Arachnidism

Bites of some spiders result in local tissue destruction and possibly systemic toxic effects. This condition has ben referred to as necrotic arachinidism. The most notorious of these spiders are those of the genus *Loxosceles*. Spiders of this genus are distributed worldwide throughout North and South America, Africa, Australia, southern Russia, as well as the Mediterranean and Orient (Gendron, 1990). *Loxosceles* spiders are fawn to dark brown in colour with relatively long skinny legs and a characteristic violin-shaped marking on their dorsal carapace (Binder, 1989). The terms brown, violin, or fiddleback spider are used to describe these species. The brown recluse spider, *Loxosceles reclusa,* is the most significant species in the USA and this has been extensively studied and exemplifies the toxicity associated with these spiders.

The diagnosis of brown recluse envenomation and its actual incidence are difficult to establish because of other potential causes of necrotic wounds, including bites of other spiders and confusing medical conditions. Such as infections or toxic epidermal necrolysis (Russell and Gertsch, 1983). Diagnostic difficulties have also hampered attempts to study promising treatment modalities. For example, in one series of 95 cases of presumed brown recluse spider bite, only 17 cases could be confirmed and ultimately studied (Rees *et al.,* 1987). A lymphocyte transformation test has been developed to aid in the diagnosis of *Loxosceles reclusa* envenomation but it is not routinely available (Berger *et al.,* 1973a).

The brown recluse spider is distributed primarily in the south-central USA (Majeski and Durst, 1976). Most reported bites have occurred in Arkansas, Kansas, Missouri and Oklahoma. These spiders inhabit primarily warm, dry, secluded places and can be found both indoors and outdoors. The household cupboard (closet) is the most frequently reported site of discovery (Rees and Campbell, 1989). Other potential sites include wood piles, storage buildings, stored clothing, attics, basements and other quiet locations. The brown recluse is nocturnal and as a result most bites occur during the night (Rees and Campbell, 1989). These spiders are most active in summer months and hibernate during the winter.

Toxic Manifestations

The venom of the brown recluse is both cytotoxic and haemolytic. Studies of the venom have identified at least nine proteins, most notably a hyaluronidase which accounts for the spreading of injected venom, and sphinogomyelinase D which likely contributes to its haemolytic and cytotoxic properties (Wasserman, 1988; Hobba and Harrell, 1989; Rees and Campbell, 1989). The quantity of injected venomis relatively small and by itself is unlikely to cause significant injury. The destructive nature of the venomis apparently facilitated by complement activation and the subsequent inflammatory response. This results in endothelial cell damage, haemorrhage, infiltration of polymorphonuclear leucocytes and thrombosis of venules and arterioles causing necrosis (Berger *et al.,* 1973b).

The bite of a brown recluse spider results in little more than a stinging or prick sensation and may go unnoticed by the victim. The clinical manifestations following envenomation depend on the amount of venom injected, the site of envenomation, and the age, underlying health and immune status of the victim (Majeski and Durst, 1976; Wasserman and Anderson, 1983-84). Not all patients develop the characteristic necrotic lesion or potentially severe systemic effects. It may be that most often only minimal envenomation results and victims experience mild discomfort that resoles within a few days (Berger, 1973).

Most patients, even following significant envenomation, do not present for treatment until many hours after the bite, once the initial signs of a necrotic lesion become evident (Gendron, 1990). The most common presenting signs and symptoms include erythema, cellulitis, generalized rash, blister pain, pruritus, malaise, chills and sweats (Rees *et al.,* 1987). The characteristic lesion begins as a blister with surrounding is chemical discolouration (Wasserman and Anderson, 1983-84; Hobbs and Harrell, 1989). An erythematous ring may surround this area giving a characteristic 'bulls eye' or 'halo' appearance (Wasserman and Anderson, 1983-84). The blister subsequently becomes a bluish macule, the centre of which generally sinks below surrounding tissue (Hobbs and Harrell, 1989). Over several days the necrotic lesion may progress resulting in an area of eschar which sloughs off after 7-14 days leaving an area of ulceration from 1 to 30 cm in diameter (Wasserman an Anderson, 1983-84; Hobbs and Harrell, 1989). Bites in fatty areas of the body tend to become more extensive (Wasserman and Anderson, 1983-84). It may take weeks to months for this area to heal by second intention. A small percentage of patients may develop persistant lesions which could subsequently progress to the development of yoderma gangrenosum and pseudoepithelomtous hyperplasia (Rees *et al.,* 1987; Hover *et al.,* 1990).

Systemic toxicity occurs less commonly and may not develop for 24-72 h after the bite. Systemic toxic effects may toxic effects may include fever, malaise, arthralgias, myalgias, rash, convulsions, haemolysis, thrombocytopenia, anaemia, and disseminated intravascular coagulation (Wasserman and Anderson, 1983-84). Nephrotoxicity may result as a complication of haemolysis and subsequent haemoglobinuria.

Management

The treatment of necrotic arachnidism, regardless of the spider involved, should consist of sound local wound management. This should include thorough cleansing, tetanus prophylaxis as necessary, immobilization, elevation and rat (Wasserman, 1988). Cool compresses may held relieve inflammation an pain (Gendronb, 1990). Prophylactic antibiotics generally are not indicated and steroid therapy has not been found to be effective (Wasserman, 1988). Symptomatic relief can be provided with the use of antipuritic, analgesic and antianxiety agents. In definite cases of brown recluse spider bite, in which there is progressive local involvement , dapsone therapy may help to limit the necrotic lesions and speed healing (Berger, 1984). It is postulated that dasponse maybe effective by reducing ploymorphonuclear leucocyte infiltration (King and Rees, 1983). Dapsone itself, however, may produce dose-dependent haemolytic anaemia, which is likely to be more severe in those with glucose-6-phosphate dehydrogenase deficiency. It should, therefore, be used cautiously and only when the diagnosis of *Loxosceles reclusa* envenomation is certain. Early excisional therapy should be avoided as it has been shown to be ineffective and potentially disfiguring or disabling (Wasserman and Anderson, 1983-84).

In cases of systemic involvement, therapy should be directed as specific complications. Systemic corticosteroids may help reduce venominduced destrutin of red blood cells. Platelests and packed red blood cells may be indicated in the presence of thrombocytopenia or anaemia, respectively. Good hydration should be maintained and renal function monitored. Alkalininzation of the urine is indicated in the presence of haemoglobinuria or haematuria.

A brown recluse spider antivenin has been prepared and has been shown *in vitro* to abolish the dermonecrotic activity of brown recluse venom (Rees *et al.*, 1984). In a clinical trial involving 17 patients antivenin was comparably effective to dapsone therapt alone or dapsone in combination with antivenin (Rees *et al.*, 1987). Further evaluation of these therapeutic approaches is warranted. The development of highly refined antivenin would be a tremendous tehrapeutic advance for brown recluse spider bites.

Scorpions

True scorpions are arachnids of the order scorpionida. There are approximately 650 species distributed worldwide, only a few of which are of significant medical importance (Currey *et al.,* 1983-84). All of these are in the Buthidae family. Scorpions primarily inhabit deserts and semi-arid regions. While scorpions are native to certain localities. It is important to recognize that they may be inadvertently transported in luggage or other goods to distant areas (Trestrail, 1981).

In the USA the most significant of all the scorpions is *Centruroides exilicauda* (bark scorpion) which is found primarily in Arizona, but also inhabits areas within New Mexico, California and Texas as well as Mexico (Likes *et al.,* 1984). A number of other scorpions which can produce significant envenomation may be found in Sought America, northern and southern Africa, India and the Middle East (Banner, 1989). Scorpions are nocturnal and take shelter during the day under rocks, piles of debris, or may hide inside house in clothing or shoes. The bark scorpion notoriously shelters under the loose bark of trees, and in crevices of dead trees or logs (Likes *et al.,* 1984). Scorpions feed primarily on insects, spiders and occasionally on other scorpions (Banner, 1989).

Scorpions have a hard skeleton and three primary body parts: the cephalothorax, to which are attached a pair of pincers; an abdomen, which has four pairs of legs; and a tail which is segmented and ends in a telson which contains the stinging apparatus. The telson contains two venom glands which lead via independent ducts to the stinger. The scorpion uses its pincers to grab its prey and then arches its tail over its body and head to inject venom. Likewise, the scorpion may grab the skin of humans and sting, sometimes repeatedly, itself-defence.

Toxic Manifestations

The venom of scorpions is primarily neurotoxic. This property appears to result from its effects on the activation and inactivation of sodium channels, which ultimately results in the release of catecholamines and acetylcholine (Wang and Strichartz, 1983; Banner, 1989). Other venom fractions exhibit enzymatic, anticholines-terase coagulupathic, haemolytic, cardiotoxic and pancreatotoxic properties (Banner, 1989).

Most envenomations occur on the extremities. Adults are most commonly stung; however, children are more likely to develop serious toxicity (Curry *et al.,* 1983-84; Likes *et al.,* 1984). This sting of *Centrulroides exilicauda* cause local pain, numbness, hyperaesthesia, salivation, agritation, wheezing, tacyycardia, hypertension and muscle spasms (Likes *et al.,* 1984). In severe cases, cranial nerve and somatic motor abnormalities such as eye movement disorders, blurred vision, tongue fasciculations, impaired pharyngeal muscle control and jerking of the extremities may develop (Curry *et al.,* 1983-84). It is notable that the bark scorpion causes few if any local effects such as inflammation or swelling. In the presence of such findings other scorpion species are the likely culprit.

Centruroides and *Titus* scorpions are of importance in South America. Neurologic toxicity is the primary concern but it is important to note that with *Titus* species parasympathetic effects predominate (Bannes; 1989). *Titus* scorpion envenomation may also produce significant local pain and erythema. This species has also been reported to produce pancreatitis (Bartholomew, 1970).

In South Africa, the most important genera of scorpions of include *Parabuthus* and *Bothotus.* These scorpions most commonly sting their victims; however, certain species of *Parabuthus* are also capable of squirting venom for up to 1 meter (Newlands, 1978). It the venom enters the eye or open wound it can cause toxicity comparable to that of the spitting cobra. Local effects following envenomation by these South African scorpions include local burning and possibly swelling. Systemic toxicity may include muscle contractions, convulsions, perspiration, salivation, tachycardia, arrhymis and irregular respirations (Newlands, 1978). Death may result from respiratory or cardiac failure.

Bed scorpion (*Buthus tamulus*) envenomation in India can cause severe toxicity and death. Excessive release of catecholamines can result in myocardial damage, arrhythmias, cardiac failure and pulmonary oedema (Alagesan *et al.*, 1977; Rajarajeswari *et al.*, 1979; Bawaskar, 1982). Other reported manifestations in both fatal and non-fatal cases include profuse sweating, mydriasis, vomiting and priapism (Bawaskar, 1982).

The Middle East and Northern Africa are inhabited with the yellow scorpion (*Leiurus quinquestriatus*) as well as *Androctonus* and *Buthus* species. The yellow scorpion also causes excessive release to catecholamins which can result in myocardial damage and congestive heart failure (Barzilyay *et al.*, 1982). Arrhythmias and pulmonary oedema have also been reported (Alagesan *et al.*, 1977; Rahav and Weiss, 1990).

Management

First aid for scorpion envenomation consist of good local wound care including thorough cleansing and tetanus prophylaxis if necessary. Cold compresses can be applied to help relieve pain and inflammation if present. Systemic manifestations of envenomation can generally be managed conservatively with traditional supportive measures. Atropine sulphate may be indicated to control excessive parasympathetic manifestations; however, this is often not necessary (Banner, 1989). Excessive adrenergic toxic effects can be controlled using adrenertgic blocking agents such as the β-antagonist propranolol or possibly the shorter acting agent esmolol (Rachesky *et al.*, 1984; Banner, 1989). Severe hypertension, unresponsive to conservative measures, may respond to intravenous hydralazine or sublingual nifedipine (Sofer and Gueron, 1990). Recent evidence further suggests that vasodilator therapy can effectively control hypertension and the cardiac sequale resulting from scorpion envenomation (Gueron and Sofer, 1990).

Antivenin therapy may have an important role in

therapy for certain scorpion envenomations. Antivenin is available in India, Israel, South Africa, North Africa and Mexico (Banner, 1989). In the USA an antivenin for *C. exilicauds* has been derived from goat serum, but it is not approved by the Food and Drug Administration (Rachesky *et al.,* 1984). It has been used safely and successfully to relieve severe signs and symptoms of envenomation; however, experience to date is limited (Curry *et al.,* 1983-84). Experience with antivenin in other parts of the world is also limited and issues relative to safety, efficacy and specificity remain to be resolved.

Jellyfish

The phylum Cnidaria (formerly Coelenterata) includes the subphylum Scyphoza, the true jellyfish. The Portuguese man-o'-war, although generally considered a jellyfish, is actually a Cnidarian of the subphylum Hydrozoa. Because of marked similarities, however, the Portuguese man-o's-war will be discussed here with the true jellyfish.

The most notable of these species are the box jellyfish (*Chironex fleckeri*), which inhabits the coastal waters of Australia and the Indo-Pacific region; the Portuguese mon-o'-war (*Physalia physalis*), located in the more tropical waters of the Atlantic; the sea nettle (*Chrysaora quinquecirrha*), which is endemic to the Chesapeake Bay and the mid-Atlantic coastal waters of the USA; and the Pacific Portuguese man-o'-war (*Physalia utriculus*), which is often responsible for stings in Hawaiian waters. Other species of jelly fish can also be found in these and other waters throughout the world.

The hanging tentacles of jellyfish contain thousands of stinging organcells known as nematocyst. Within the nematocyst is a coiled threadlike structure coated with venom. In response to pressure or changes in osmolarity the nematocyst fires its thread which can penetrate the skin to cause envenomation.

The venom of jellyfish contains various polypeptides and enzymes. It is in both toxic and allergenic. In animal studies the venom has been shown to produce dermonecrosis, vasopermeability, haemolysis, cardiotoxicity, neurotoxicity, musculotoxicity and cytotoxicity. A kinin-like fraction has also been identified which is believed to account for pain.

Toxic Manifestations

The most common manifestations from Cnidaria envenomation are local toxic effects. Severe systemic and allergic reactions, as well as delayed or recurrent dermal effects also may occur. The severity of envenomation is dependent on a number of factors including the species of jellyfish, the extent and duration of contact with tentacles and the resultant number of fired nematocysts, the amount of venom available in the nematocyst at the time of firing, the thickness of the skin, and the size, age and underlying health of the victim.

Dermal contact with jellyfish tentacles typically results in linear, urticarial and painful eruptions which are the result of toxic effects of the venom. The sting of the Portuguese man-o'-war is generally considered more painful than that of the sea nettle, and the local pain from envenomation by the box jellyfish can be excruciating. The resultant lesions may be vesicular, haemorrhagic, necrotizing or ulcerative (Burnett *et al.,* 1987a). Subacute or chronic reactions may include localized hyperhidrosis, desquamation, lymphadenopathy, angiooedma, urticaria, keloid formation, hyper-or hypopigmentation, local fat atrophy, contractions, vasospasm, gangrene and nerve damage (Burnett and Calton, 1987b; Burnett *et al.,* 1987a).

An allergic response may contribute to the local effects. In fact, a large local reaction comparable to that seen with hymenoptera stings has been described. Recurrent eruptions at the site of the initial sting and at distant sites have also been reported. It has been postulated that an antigen depot must exist for this to occur. There is also evidence that individuals may crossreact with different animals of this phylum. The potential for an an aphylactoid reaction must be considered.

Jellyfish envenomation may result in severe systemic toxic reactions and even death. The most common systemic toxic effects include headache, nausea, vomiting, malaise, weakness, perspiration and lachrymation (Burnett *et al.*, 1987a). More severe manifestations include hypotension, cardiac conduction disturbances, arrhythmias, respiratory depression, pulmonary oedema and cardiovascular collapse.

Death from jellyfish envenomation may result from either allergic or toxic mechanisms. The box jellyfish is the most toxic of all marine animals and has been implicated in most jellyfish related fatalities. It is not clear whether death results from cardiotoxicity or respiratory failure.

Management

Victims of jellyfish envenomation should be kept quiet and the affected limb should be immobilized because muscle activity may increase the firing of nematocysts. The exposed a area should be rinsed with sea water. Fresh water is contraindictated as this too will increase nematocyst firing as a result of osmotic changes. The next step is to inactivate the nematocysts which is a species-specific process. For most species this can be accomplished by flooding the area with household vinegar (5 per cent acetic acid). In the event of sea nettle or lion's mane jellyfish envenomation a baking soda slurry is more appropriate (Burnett and Calton, 1987b). Nematocysts can then be removed from the skin by scraping with a blunt edged object such as a sea shell, credit card or by shaving with a razor. Application of a cold pack may help relieve mild to moderate pain (Exton *et al.*, 1989). Topical anaesthe-tics or steroid creams as well as oral analgesics may benefit some patients. Hyperpigement action can be treated with bleaching a agent such as tropical hydroquinone.

Systemic manifestations are managed with traditions supportive measures. The calcium channel antagonist verapamil hydrochloride has been shown to inhibiting the action of box jellyfish cardiotoxin and prolong survival in mice. This finding has been extended to other jellyfish species. It is, therefore, recommended that patients who manifest cardiac dysfunction should be treated with verpamil. An antivenin is available for the box jellyfish from the Commonwealth Serum Laboratory in Melbourne, Australia.

Anithistamines may be useful if there is evidence of all an allergic response to the venom. Anaphylactoid reactions reactions should be managed accordingly. In the event of recurrent dermal eruptions a tapering dose of a corticosteriod may be employed.

In addition to the Portuguese man-o'-war another important Hydrozoan is fire coral. The fire coral, while not a true coral, is so named because of its marked resemblance to these species. Polyps which contain nematocysts protrude through pores of its calcareous skeleton. It typically produces only mild dermatitis and burning discomfort (Kizer, 1983-84). The subphylum anthosa includes the sea anemones which also contain modified nematocysts capable of inflicting stings and local effects as described for the cnidarjans.

Stingrays

Another important coastal hazard is the stingray. Approximately 20 species have been described (Fenner *et al.,* 1989). These creatures are often found partially buried in the sand and are a significant hazard to beachcombers and to those who swim or play in shallow water. Although normally very docile, stingrays will lash their tails forward and sting with a spine located near the base of the tail if they are stepped on or otherwise abruptly disturbed. Some species of stingray contain more than one spine and are capable of inflicting multiple simultaneous stings.

The stinging spine(s) of stingrays are covered by a venom-containing integumentary sheath. As the spine enters the victim this sheath may rupture resulting in the release of venom into the wound. The spines of stingrays very by species and may range from 2.5 cm to 12 mm in length. The spine is curved and serrated enabling it to inflict significant trauma in addition to envenomating the victim. A large stingray, in fact, is capable of inflicting fatal traumatic injury.

Toxic Manifestations

Most stings are to the lower extremities (Russell *et al.,* 1958). The upper extremities, abdomen or thorax may be involved from careless handling or under extraordinary circumstances. The stingray's venom consists of a heat-labile protein that causes intense pain at the site of sting which is out of proportion to the physical trauma. In the event that the wound is not characteristically painful and other toxic manifestations do not occur it is likely that the integumentary sheth had already been lost or it was not disrupted during the sting. The venom can produce local tissue necrosis which complicates the healing process (Fenner *et al.,* 1989). It has also been shown in animal models to possess both cardiotoxic and neurotoxic properties (Russell *et al.,* 1958). Systemic manifestations from envenomation may include nausea; vomiting, diarrhoea; salivation, generalized oedema; headache; vertigo; syncope; respiratory depression and distress; cardiac conduction disturbances and arrhythmias; hypotension, muscle cramps, fasciculations, tremor and seizures; and death. Secondary infections are also possible.

Management

First aid for stingray envenomation consists of washing the wound with sea water and as soon as possible soaking he site in water that is as hot as the patient can tolerate for 30-90 min to denature the thermolabile venom (Russell *et al.,* 1958; Fenner *et al.,* 1989). The wound should then be surgically explored to remove any remaining fragments of the sheath or spine. Necrotic tissue should be debrided and an antiseptic should be used to cleanse the wound, which should be left open to heal by second intention. Tetanus immunization status should be updated if necessary and prophylactic antibiotics should be administered in serious cases (Fenner *et al.,* 1989). Narcotic analgesics may be necessary to control pain. No antivenin is available and systemic manifestations should be managed with traditional symptomatic and supportive care.

Stinging Fishes

Other venmous underwater creatures include fresh an salt water fishes. Common examples include the lionfish, scorpion fish, stone fish, catfish and weaver fish. All these fish sting with venomous spines associated with their fins. The sting of these fish is much less traumatic than that associated with the stingray but in other respects their stings are quite comparable. Fish stings may be inflicted in those who swim or recreate in the oceans, seas or lakes; in those who fish for recreation or commercially; and in hobbyists who may keep a venomous species in their aquaria. The lionfish is popular with salt water aquarists and has been responsible for many stings to the hand and fingers (Kizer *et al.*, 1985; Trestrail and Al-Mahasneh, 1989).

Toxic Manifestations

Fish stings result in an initial sharp stabbing pain when the spine penetrates the skin. In some cases the spine may break free and remain lodged in the wound. Severe pain may ensue which can radiate to involve the entire extremity. The pain may be excruciating and incapacitating in some cases. Pronounced local swelling occurs commonly and vesicles may form at the puncture sites (Auerbach *et al.,* 1987). The vesicular fluid may itself be harmful and prompt drainage of the fluid is recommended.

Systemic manifestations may occur with significant envenomation resulting from multiple stings or single stings from certain species such as the stone fish. These toxic effects may include nausea, vomiting, diaphoresis, bradycardia or tachcardia, conduction disturbances, hypotension, myocardial ischaemia, respiratory distress, muscle tremor, weakness, delirium, convulsions and death (Kizer *et al.,* 1985; Ell and Yates, 1989).

Management

As with the stingray the venom of these fish consists primarily of a heat labile protein. Accordingly, first aid treatment should include immersion of the affected site in water as hot as the patient can tolerate for 30-90 min. Afterwards the site should be thoroughly cleaned and in some cases the wound may need to be surgically explored to remove any remaining spine. Tetanus prophylazxis should be updated as necessary. Prophylactic antinbiotics are not routinely necessary. It is important to recognize that failure to treat these inflictions promptly may result in permanent scaring and physical impairment. Systemic manifestations should be managed with traditional supportive and symptomatic measures. An antivenin is available for the management of stone fish envenomation.

Poisonous Fish and Shellfish

In addition to those animals that can cause human poisoning by envenomation, several toxic syndromes may results from ingestion of various fish and shellfish. In some cases these animals excrete the toxin, but most concentrate toxins that are produced by dinoflagellates or bacteria. Fish can be categorized based on the tissue that contains the toxin (Halstead, 1964). Ichthyosarcotoxic fish, which cause most poisoning, have toxin in muscle, viscera, skin or mucus. Ichthyootoxic fish produce toxin concentrated in the gonads. Ichthyohaemotoxic fish, which rarely produce poisoning, have toxin in their blood. Toxic syndromes resulting from ingestion of poisonous aquatic life are unlike traditional food poisoning which is associated with ingestion of microbial contaminated foods.

Ciguatera Fish Poisoning

Citguatera intoxication is the most common type of ichthyvosarcotoxic fish poisoning. The primary responsible toxin ciguatoxin, is produced by the dinoflagellate *Gambierdiscus toxicus* (Eastaugh and Shephered, 1989). Although it has anticholinesterase activity, its primary mechanism of action is thought to be from competitive inhibition of calcium-regulated sodium channels (Eastaugh and Shephered, 1989). Ciguatoxin a heat-stable, lipid-soluble compound that is resistant to gastric acid (Estaugh and Shepherd, 1989). It can be excreted in breast milk which can cause toxicity in nursing infants (Blythe and deSylva, 1990). Maitotoxin, scaritoxin, lysophosphatidylcholine, ATPase inhibitor and possibly an indole-positive toxin may also contribute to toxicity (Sims, 1987). Toxins are concentrated up the food chain; as a result large fish are most likely to cause human poisoning. Hundreds of fish species have been reported to harbour ciguatoxin; common examples include the barracuda, grouper, snapper, amberjack and sea bass (Halstead, 1964).

Most outbreaks of ciguatera intoxication occur in the Caribbean and South Pacific. In the USA most cases have been reported in Hawaii and Florida (Hughes and Merson, 1976). Ciguatera poisoning, however, has also been associated with ingestion of fish caught from the southeastern USA coastal waters as far as north as North Carolina (Morris *et al.,* 1990). The ability readily to transport fish great distances may result in ciguatera poisoning in virtually any geographic region. People of Chinese or Philippine descent are likely to be more severely affected but Hawaiians least affected (Sims, 1987). This ethni variation is not well understood.

Toxic Manifestation

Ciguatera poisoning affects primarily the gastrointestinal and nervous systems. Signs and symptoms usually develop within 6 h; however, there is considerable variability. Common gastrointestinal effects include diarrhoea, vomiting and abdominal pain (Morris *et al.,* 1982). These symptoms generally occur early resolve within 24 h. Other initial symptoms may include malaise, pain and weakness in the lower extremities, dysaesthesias including reversal of hot and cold sensation, and paraesthesias around the mouth and of the extremities (Hughes and Merson, 1976; Morris *et al.,* 1982). These effects may persist for weeks or months. Other common findings include rash, dry mouth, metallic taste, myalgias, arthralgia, visual disturbances and a sensation of loose teeth. Bradycardia, hypotension and respiratory paralysis may occur in severe cases (Hughes and Merson, 1976).

Management

Gastointestinal decontamination may be helpful if the toxic nature of the fish is recognized soon after ingestion. Treatment is primarily symptomatic and supportive care. Fluid and electrolyte balance should be monitored as well as the electrocardiogram. Atropine and intravenous fluids have been effective in the treatment of bradycardia and hypotension. Mannitol was found to improve neurological and gastrointestinal toxicity dramatically in a group of 24 patients (Palafox *et al.,* 1988). It is postulated that mannitol may have inactivated the toxin or competitively inhibited its action on the sodium channel.

Paralytic Shellfish Poisoning

Paralytic shellfish poisoning result from ingestion of contaminated bivalve molluscs such a clams and oysters. These molluscs concentrate neurotoxins known as saxitoxins, which are produced by a number of dinoflgellates including those of the *Gonyaulax* and *Pyridinum* species (Eastaugh and Shepherd, 1989; Rodrigue *et al.,* 1990). The toxin is water soluble, heat and acid stable compound which cannot be destroyed by ordinary cooking (Auerbach and Halstead, 1989). The toxin acts by interfering with sodium conductance thereby inhibiting neuromuscular transmission.

Toxic Manifestations

As the name implies, paralytic shellfish poisoning primarily affects the nervous system. Prominent toxic effects include paraesthesias of the lips, face and extremities; headache, weakness; dizziness; vertigo; and difficulty walking (Hughes and Merson, 1976; Eastaugh and Shepherd, 1989). A sensation of floating has also been described (McColloum *et al.,* 1968). In the severe cases muscle paralysis may occur. Death may result from respiratory arrest if adequate life-support cannot be provided. Some neurological symptom such as headaches, memory loss and fatigue may persist for up to 2 weeks (Rodrigue *et al.,* 1990).

Management

Astrointestinal decontamination should be performed if the toxic nature of the mollusc is recognized soon after consumption. The remainder of therapy is basically symptomatic and supportive care. Respiratory function should be monitored closely with ventilatory assistance provided as needed.

Neurotoxic Shellfish Poisoning

A milder introxication, known as neurotoxic shellfish poisoning, may result from ingestation of contaminated shellfish off the western Florida coast of the USA (Sakamoto *et al.,* 1987). The toxins, brevitoxins, from the dinoflagellate *Ptychodiscus brevis* stimulate postganglionic cholinergic nerve fibers (Graunfeld and Spiegeslstein, 1974; Asai *et al.,* 1982). Toxic manifestations include nausea, vomiting, diarrhoea and paraesthesias. As with ciguatera poisoning, patient may experience the hot-cold reversal phenomenon (Hughes and Meson, 1976; Sims, 1987).

Domoic Acid Intoxication

A unique toxic syndrome was recently described that resulted from ingestion of contaminated mussels from Prince Edward Island in Canada (Perl *et al.,* 1990). Domoic acid was implicated as the responsible toxin, which was apparently produced by the marine algae *Nitzschia pungens.* Domoic acid is an excitatory neurotransmitter structually similar to glutamic acid and kainic acid (Teitelbaum *et al.,* 1990).

The most common acute symptom of intoxication included causes, vomiting, abdominal cramps, diarrhoea, headache and memory loss (Perl *et al.,* 1990). In severe cases altered mental status, seizures, myoclonus and cardiovascular instability resulted. Death was reported in four cases. The initial widespread neurotoxicity and subsequent chronic residual memory impairment differentiates this syndrome from either paralytic or neurotoxic shellfish poisoning.

Tetrodotoxic Fish Poisoning

Tetrodotoxication is primarily associated with ingestion of the puffer fish and relate fish of the order Tetraodontiformes. Other animals also may contain this neurotoxin, for example the Californian newt (*Taricha torosa*), Pacific goby (*Gobius criniger*), and Costa Rican frog (Tibballs, 1988).

Tetrodotoxin acts similar to saxitoxin in that it blocks neurotransmission by action on sodium channels. This results in motor, autonomic and sensory nerve impairment (Tibballs, 1988). It also has direct action on the medulla, stimulating the chemoreceptor trigger zone and depressing the respiratory center (Eastaugh and Shepherd, 1989).

Toxic Manifestations

Prominent signs and symptoms of introxication include persistent vomiting, paraesthesias, weakness, respiratory impairment, hypotension and breadycardia. Other manifestation may include headache, dilated pupils, salivation, diaphoresis, myalgias, dysarthria, ataxia, muscle fasciculations and seizures. Death may results in severe cases from respiratory failure or cardivascular collapse.

Management

Treatment is primarily sympomatic and supportive care. Gastric lavage should be performed if it can be done after ingestion. Activated charcoal is also recommended. Ventilatory assistance maybe required in sever cases Hypotension and bradycardia should be managed with atropine and fluid therapy. Vasopressors, such as do amine hydrochloride, may be required.

Scombroid Fish Poisoning

Scombroid fish poisoning is a toxic syndrome that

resembles an acute allergic reaction. It results from ingestion of spoiled fish that is contaminated with histamine and possibly other toxins. Histamine is formed as a result of bacteria that cause enzymatic decarboxylation of histidine, which is normally present in the flesh of certain fish species (Lerke *et al.,* 1978). Fish most commonly involved are those of the suborder *scombroidei* such as the tuna, mackerel, bonito, skipjack and saury. Other marine fish such as the mahimahi have also been implicated in outbreaks of scombroid intoxication (Eastaugh and Shepherd, 1989).

The association between histamine and scombrid intoxication is unclear. Histamine has limited activity when administered orally because of rapid metabolism and elimination in the urine (Garrison, 1990). This evidence and the effectiveness of antihistamines to relieve symptoms of scombroid intoxication implicate histamine as the causative toxin. Other substances in spoiled fish such as cadaverine or putrescine might histamine-metabolizing enzymes, thereby allowing the absorption of histamine (Auerbach, 1990). This is an area that warrants further investigation.

Toxic Manifestations

Scokbroid intoxication usually results in a relatively mild, self-limited syndrome, which usually begins within 1 h of ingestion and lasts for 8 h or less (Merson *et al.,* 1974; Hughes and Meson, 1976). Typical manifestations include nausea, diarrhoea, abdominal cramps, vomiting, throbbing headache, oral blistering or burning sensation, flushing, burning sensation of the skin , and urticaria. Tachycardia, palpitations, bronochospasm and respiratory distess may also occur (Merson *et al.,* 1974; Hughes and Merson, 1976; Blakesley, 1983).

Management

Treatment is primarily symptomatic and supportive care. If the fish is recognized as poisonous soon after ingestion the gastrointestinal tract should be decontaminated. Antihistamines such as diphenhydramine are the mainstay of therapy. The use of cimetidine in few cases has been shown to dramatically relieve the signs and symptoms of scombroid intoxication. Bronchodilators may be needed in the event of bronchospasm.

It is important to differentiate between scombroid poisoning and fish allergy. An incorrect diagnosis of fish allergy will unnecessarily limit the diet of the patient. Considerations include the patient's prior to ingestion of the implicated fish species and the response in others who consumed the same meal. The food can be analysed for the presence of histamine but at this time there are no diagnostic tests that can be performed on the patient.

Acknowledgements

The author acknowledges the careful and critical review of this chapter by David E. Seidler, MD, Kay A. Wallander, PharmD, and Lynn F. Durback, RN, BSN, CSPI and the expert technical assistance of Tina C. Means.

10

Radiation Toxicology

Introduction

Ionizing radiation caused many different types of damage in mammalian systems. These include effects in both prolierative and non-proliferative tissues, the induction of genetic abnormalities that in some circumstances can be passed on to offspring, and the induction of malignancy. The nature and severity of radiation-induced effects can vary with radiation type; the magnitude of the radiation dose and the period over which it is delivered; the age, sex, and health status of the individual; and particularly, the degree of post-irradiation care that may be available.

The energies of radiation emanating from X-ray sets, many radionuclides and particle accelerators are usually vastly in excess of the chemical bonds that are present in all biological molecules. Following interaction between radiation and any molecule, simple or complex, electron ejecting, or ionizatink is the primary event. The time-scale is governed by various factors, but a quantum of gamma-radiation or a high-energy particle will pass through a small molecule and impart energy to it in times of the order of 10^{-17}s. The subsequent physical, chemical and biological processes are complex and occur over very different time-scales. For example, the onset of malignancy does not occur in many instances until 20 or even 30 years after irradiation.

It is often convenient, though not necessarily rigorous to classify radiation action into physical, chemical, cellular, and tissue effects.

The Physical and Chemical Stages

Radiation deposits energy in discrete packages in 'tracks' through the absorbing medium. Thee spatial distribution of energy deposition depends on the type of radiation, the composition of the medium and the energy of the radiation. The so-called densely ionizing radiations such as α-particles, neutrons and heavier particles, lose energy over much shorter distances than low linear energy transfer (LET) radiations such as X- or y-rays. LET is a measure of the rate at which energy is imparted to the absorbing medium per unit distance of track length. The biological effectiveness of the former type is generally greater in inducing most types of biological effect, including malignancy. Particulate radiations, with the exception of neutrons, are absorbed over short distances, except at extremely high energies. Following primary ionizations, the secondary electrons, which are still highly energietic lose enegy by various collisional and othe inteactions, thereby producing other ions, excited molecules and molecular fragments.

The chemical stage of radiation action is mainly concerned with the formation , diffusion and eventual reaction of the molecular fragments and other unstable initiates. Because of the high energy of the radiations relative to the normal bond energies in molecules, radiation is absorbed fairly non-selectively. This is not necessarily true in all cases, particularly in materials abundant in heavy atoms, but it is certainly a sound approximation in biological material. The 'principle of equipartition of energy' implies that, in cellular material about 80 per cent of the energy is initially deposited in the aqueous component. This is way so much attention has been given in the past to the study of the radiation chemistry of water—particularly, aqueous solutions or mixtures containing various biological molecules. There is now abundant evidence that damage to such molecules, particularly the nucleic acids, caused by free radicals, contributes to loss or change of intercellular function following irradiation. The continuing problem however, is to distinguish those processes that are relevant to the observed cellular response to radiation from those that are not.

The Cellular Stage

Various morphological changes in the cell can often be observed shortly after irradiation. Local protrusion of the plasma membrane follow within minutes of exposure to relatively high doses of radiation. These are followed within hours by other membrane changes including an increase in permeability and loss of essential enzymes. However, the more-important effects concerning the loss of, or changes in cellular function that occur at much lower doses can only be observed much later. For clonogenic cells *in vitro,* loss of reproductive capacity is evident only when the cells fail to divide. Subcellular effects, such as mutation and the induction of aberrant chromosomes, can only be observed when sufficient cell divisions have take place to permit analysis. Mammalian cells are often at their most sensitive during mitosis and early in G phase. Resistance is usually great during early S phase, although this is very dependent on radiation quality, i.e., the type of radiation.

Repair processes occur in irradiated cells both *in vitro* and *in vivo.* When radiation is delivered at a low dose rate or in a series of multiple fractions separated by several hours, the overall effect on cell-kill is usually less than for an acute dose of radiation. This phenomenon, more commonly seen with low LET radiation, is attributable to repair of sublethal injury. It is relevant to dose-response relationships for cell-kill and various sublethal effects such as mutation and cell transformation. Repair processes of various kinds occur both *in vitro* and *in vivo* and are responsible for the reduced severity of some radiation injuries when the exposure is protracted.

Radiation dose to tissue is expressed in terms of the quantity of absorbed energy per unit mass. The SI unit is the gray (Gy), which id defined as 1 joule of absorbed energy per kilogram. The older unit, the rad, which is till in common use, is equivalent to 100 erg g^{-1} and equal to 0.01; Gy. A dose of G of X-rays will cause about 2×10^5 separate ionizations within the mammalian cell. Of these, about 1 per cent occur in the genomic material and a major consequence of this is breakage of DNA strands. Of the many breaks that occur, almost all disappear within a few hours, probably by enzyme-mediated repair. Some breaks remain, however, probably as aligned double-strand breaks, and these are the major cause of loss of cell viability and also contributed to various type so sublethal injury. In many mammalian cells it is remarkable that, for this high dose of radiation, a substantial population of the cells retain a degree of reproductive capacity despite the large amount of chemical damage sustained by the cells. Much of the initial chemical damage caused by the radiation must therefore to be little consequence to the fate of the cell. It is likely that only a small part of the damage, caused perhaps by the rather rare local deposition of energy close to critical molecular sites in important.

The Tissue Stage

The response time of mammalian tissues to radiation varies widely, as do their sensitivities. The general finding *in vitro* that mammalian cells are at their most radiation-sensitive during mitosis predicts that *in vivo* the mammalian fertilized egg cell (zygote) will be highly radiation-sensitive and that tissues with high rates of cell turnover will also be particularly sensitive. Both predictions are correct. Rapidly proliferating stem cells of the intestinal epithelium and the haematopoietic system are highly sensitive and respond more rapidly than do less sensitive cells, such as those in the lung and the basal layer of the skin, which have lower proliferation rates. Cells that do not divide, or do son only after an appropriate stimulus, e.g., parenchymal cells of the liver, are less sensitive still. Cell that divide only during embryogenesis are the least sensitive.

In this chapter the nature, origin and expression of radiation injury are classified according to the organ in which it occurs, and particularly with regard to the stockhastic or nonstochastic nature of the pathological response. The International Commission on Radiological Protection (ICRP) made the distinction between stochastic and non-stochastic effects (ICRP, 1977). Stochastic effects are those for which the probability of an effect occurring, but not its severity, increases with radiation dose, without a threshold. In contrast, non-stockhastic effects are those for which the severity of the effect depends on the magnitude of the dose, and for which a threshold exists, below which no detrimental effects are observable. The types of damage that result from injury to substantial population of cells in tissues such as the eye, skin, lung, gonads, gastrointestinal tract and haematopoietic system are considered to be non-stochastic. On the other hand, stockastic effects can result from injury to a single cell or to a small number of cells, and include the induction of various hereditary defects an most types of cancer.

A further distinctions often made between the somatic and hereditary effects of radiation. Somatic effects refer to those which are manifest in the exposed individual, and include both non-stochastic and stochastic effects. The hereditary effects of radiation are of a stochastic nature and are transmitted via germ cell damage. The effects may be expressed in the immediate offspring or in later generations.

Non-Stochastic Effects

Non-stockhastic radiation effects are due to radiation-induced cell killing with the accompanying disruption of functions for which the cells are responsible.

Cell death is most likely to occur when the irradiated cell attempts to resume dividing. This leads to lack of replacement of mature cells which have been lost through natural senescence and death. For certain cell types, including lymphocytes and ocytes, radiation-induced cell death occurs during interphase. In general, the rate at which cells divide, differentiate, age and are lost from a given tissue will influence the rapidity with which that tissue exhibits radiation damage. Those tissues containing actively dividing cells will tend to exhibit greater radiosensitivity than do those composed of fully differentiated cells with little or no mitotic activity.

The life-span of the comparatively radioresistant mature cells represents a further factor influencing the interval between irradiation and the time when damage becomes evident in tissues with well-defined stem cell population. In the case of fractionated or protracted exposures, stem cell division can partially compensate for cell killing and so reduce the effectiveness of the radiation.

Populations containing cells with a relatively short life-span, e.g. the gastrointestinal mucosa, will exhibit radiation damage much more quickly than populations where the cell life-span is longer, e.g. blood cells of the circulatory system. On this basis it is possible to distinguish between early effects, which may appear within a few weeks, depending on the pattern of exposure, and later effects, which do not appear until months or years after irradiation.

In those tissues which lack a well-define stem cell population and exhibit low cellular proliferations, radiation effects, although does-dependent, any not appear for some time. These tissues, e.g. the liver, where the turnover of parenchymal cells is low, have much less protection from the effects of radiation in the absence of an ability to compensate for cell killing through stem cell proliferation.

Other factors, besides the proliferative ability of cells in a given tissue, which may contribute to a reduction in effects of irradiation include tissue repopulation by surviving cells, the ability of differentiating, maturing and functioning cells to buffer stem cell damage; the ability of a tissue to undergo compensatory changes to maintain the supply of differentiated cells; and the tissue's functional reserve capacity.

The severity and clinical expression of non-stochastic effects will differ, depending on whether an individual has received a partial or whole-body irradiation. Whole-body exposures at doses of between a few and tens of grays of acute irradiation, i.e. delivered over a short time-interval, may result in the development of the haematopoietic, gastrointestinal or cerebral syndromes. Partial-body irradiation at sufficiently high doses may result in damage to self-renewing tissues, including the skin and skin adnexa, bone marrow, gastrointestinal lining, testis and lens of the eye, and to other radiosensitive tissues, including the ovary, lung, central nervous system and kidney. Specific functioning in each of these tissues if impaired, owing to the radiation-induced loss of parenchymal cells. To some extent damage may persist even after repair and repopulation, due to the relative increase in connective tissue. This may lead to tissue fibrosis following the loss of parenchymal cells and associated functions.

In the following paragraphs the non-stochastic effects resulting from whole and partial body irradiation are considered in detail. Subsequently the stochastic effects—namely radiation carcinogenesis ad hereditary defects are—examined. The effects resulting from *in utero* irradiation are also discussed, although these are not easily classified as stochastic or nonstochastic.

Whole-body Irradiation

In man death may occur within a few weeks following acute radiation exposure. The survival time and mode of death is dose-dependent. A dose of 100 Gy can cause death from neurological damage within a few hours; 5-12 Gy can cause death from gastrointestinal injury within a few days; while 2.5-5 Gy may death from irreveribile damage to the haematopoietic system in several weeks. The prodromal syndrome develops shortly after irradiation, and precedes the onset of neurological, gastrointestinal and haemato-poietic syndromes. Although the exact cause of death in the neurological syndrome is uncertain, depletion of the stem cells in the critical self-renewing tissues of the gut epithelium and circulating blood cells causes death in the gastrointestinal and haematopoietic syndromes, respectively. Differences in the population kinetics of the gut epithelium and haematopoietic system, and the amount of damage that can be tolerated by each before death, are responsible for differences in the doses at which death occurs, and for different times of onset.

The Prodromal Syndrome

The prodormal syndrome comprises the symptoms and signs that appear within 48 h of irradiation. It is mediated through the autonomic nervous system, and appears as gastrointestinal and neuromuscular symptoms. After an acute dose of 4-5 Gy the principle symptoms include anorexia, nausesa, vomiting and fatigue. At higher doses the symptoms include diarrhoea, fever, sweating, listlessness, headache and apathy. Vomiting is infrequent at doses below 1 Gy. Prodromal symptoms may occur within an hour or so following irradiation, persist for a few days and then gradually diminish in intensity.

The Haematopoietic Syndrome

Uniform whole-body irradiation with 1-10 Gy oflow-LET radiation causes damage to he haematopoietic system. proliferating haematopoietic stem cells are highly radiosensitive and are sterilized by radiation, thereby reducing the body's supply of red and white cells and platelets. The full effect of the damage is not experienced until the number of circulating cells in the blood reachers a critical minimum value.

In human bone marrow the total number of nucleated cells is reduced at day 1 by 10-20 per cent after 1-2 Gy by 25-30 per cent after 3-4 Gy, by 50-60 per cent after 5–7 Gy and by a maximum of 80–85 percent after 8–10 Gy. Resistant cells such as macrophages, stromal cells, cells of the vascular epithelium and some mature granulocytes and eosinophils remain (IAEA, 1971).

The lymphocyte count is themost sensitive index of radiation injury in the blood; for a given dose nadir levels are reached earlier than for other cell types. Lymphocytes undergo interphase death and their numbers decrease to about 50 per cent of normal by 48 h following a dose of 1–2 Gy.

Neutrophils show an initial increase over the first few days after irradiation, then a dose-related fall. Between 10 and 15 days after a dose of 2–5 Gy, there is a second abortive rise due to recovering haematopoiesis from precursor cell populations, followed by a second decline to about day 25. This is due to a lack of recovery in the stem cell population. With doses greater than 5 Gy the second abortive rise dose not occur. The time-course for platelet loss is similar to that for granulocytes, but there is no second abortive rise. A decrease in platelet levels in the blood is associated with bleeding. Owing to the long life-span or radioresistant red blood cells (109–127 days in man), anaemia results only when there has been substantial bleeding.

Figure 2 shows data from accident cases, depicting the average time-courses for suppression and recovery of neutrophils, lymphocytes and platelets in man following irradiation.

Approximately 3 weeks after irradiation, symptoms including chills, fatigue, ulceration of the mouth and petechial haemorrhages of the skin develop as a result of the reduction in blood cells components. Infections and fever arise as a result of granulocyte depression and impairment of the immune system, while bleeding and possibly anaemia may develop from haemorrhage caused through platelet depression. Death, which is often caused by infection, will follow at this stage unless bone marrow regeneration has commenced. Where the radiation dose is less than 4–5 Gy, it is possible to treat the individual in response to specific symptoms—for example, by administering antibiotics for infection until the immune system has fully recovered.

Human develop signs of haematological damage and recover from it much more slowly than do other mammals.

Peak incidence of death occurs may continue for up to 60 days. The 50 per dent lethal dose or LD_{50} for man is therefore expressed as the $LD_{50/60}$ (i.e. the dose that caused 50 per cent mortality within 60 days), in contrast to the $LD_{50/30}$ for most animal species, where the peak incidence of death occurs between 10 and 15 days after irradiation.

The Gastrointestinal Syndrome

A whole-body dose of 10 Gy or more of low-Let radiation will produce the gastrointestinal syndrome in most mammals, resulting in death 3-10 days later. Signs and symptoms follow those of the prodromal phase, and include nausea, vomiting, increased lethargy, prolonged diarrhoea, loss of appetite, and loss of fluids and electrolytes. After a few days individuals show signs of dehydration; weight loss; gastric retention and decreased intestinal absorption; emaciation; an complete exhaustion. There is a marked reduction in the leucocyte count, and haemorrhages and bactermia may occur, aggravating the injury and contributing to death. The symptoms and subsequent death are due to the radiation-induced damage to the epithelium lining the gastrointestinal tract. A dose of about 10 Gy will sterilize a large proportion of the mitotic cells in the crypts of the intestinal mucosa. This arrests the continuous supply of new cells which normally move up the villi, differentiate to become functioning cells and eventually slough off. Sterilization of cells in the crypts prevents repopulation. After a few days, the villi began to shrink and the intestinal lining is eventually denuded to villi.

The Neurological Syndrome

A radiation dose of more than about 100 Gy will cause death from cerebrovascular damage in most mammalian species within 2 days. The neurological syndrome is characterized by severe prodromal effects followed by transitory periods of depressed or enhanced motor activity. Severe nausea may occur within minutes, which is then followed by vomiting, disorientation, loss of coordination and muscular movement, respiratory distress, diarrhoea, convulsive seizures, coma and eventually death.

The exact cause of death in the neurological syndromes is not fully understood. Although death is usually attributed to direct damage to the central nervous system, much higher doses are required to produce death if only the head is irradiated, which indicates that effects elsewhere in the body are also important . An increase in the fluid content of the brain due to leakage from small vessels creating a build-up of pressure inside has been suggested as the cause of immediate death.

Effects from Partial Body Irradiation

The lens of the eye is one of the most radiosensitive tissues of the body. Exposure to ionizing radiation may cause a cataract, a term used to describe any detectable change in the normally transparent lens of the eye. This may range from tiny flects in the lens to virtually complete pacification, causing blindness.

Radiation-induced cataracts arise through damage to the mitotic cells in the anterior epithelium of the lens. Under normal conditions these cells continue to proliferate throughout life and differentiate into lens fibres. Damage to the dividing cells results in abnormal lens fibres which are to translucent. These damaged cell and their breakdown products migrate posteriorly and accumulate beneath the capsule at the posterior pole of the lens, where they cause posterior displacement of the lens bow. If enough damaged cells accumulate, they become visible pthalomologically as a dot, usually situated at the posterior pole.

During the early stages, radiation-induced cataracts are unique in that, unlike other radiation-induced effects, they can be distinguished in most cases from cataracts resulting from other causes. As the cataract enlarges, small granules and vacuoles appear around it, and by the time the opacity is a few millimetres in diameter, it may have developed a clear centre and have assumed a doughnut shape. The radiation dose received will determine whether the cataract remains stationary or continues to progress. If the cataract progresses, it becomes indistinguishable from other types of cataract.

In human lens opacities may appear between 6 months and 35 years after irradiation. The latent period between irradiation and appearance of a cataract is dose-related. At high doses lens opacities develop within months, progress rapidly and produce vision-impairing cataracts. At lower doses the opacities develop more slowly, remain microscopic in size and cause no significant impairment of vision. A threshold dose of about 2 Gy X-irradiation in a single exposure is required for the induction of minimally detectable lens opacities; larger doses are required with fractionated or protracted exposures. Compared with the lens, other parts of the eye are less radiosensitive.

Skin

The effect of radiation on the skin is dependent on various factors, including dose, the depth and area of skin irradiated, and the anatomical locations and its vascularity. It is also influenced by the age, hormonal status and genetic background of the irradiated individual. Within hours of irradiation, transitory erythema may occur, indicating capillary dilation brought about by the release of histaminel-like substances from injured epithelial cell. Typically this persists for only a few hours. Two of four weeks later, one or more waves of deeper and more prolonged erythema usually appear. Thereafter, depending on the dose received, epilation, dry desquatmation, moist desquamation and necrosis of the skin may occur.

The severity of the skin response is determined by the dose to the germinal cell is the basal layer of the epidermis. Since damage to these cells appears to be critical to the pathogenesis of erythema and desquamation, post-irradiation treatments using corticosteroids may decrease the severity of the desquamaion reaction but will have no effect on erythema. In human skin the threshold dose of X- or gamma-rays required to produce erythema in a 10 cm^2

field range from 6-8 Gy for single, brief exposures to more than 30 Gy for highly fractionated or protracted exposures. Threshold doses for dry desquamation, moist desquatmation and necrosis are higher, but also increase with fractionated or protracted exposure.

The effect of radiation-induced damage to the dermis appears later than dose that to the epidermic or to the epidermal associated hair follicles, principally because of the slower turnover of cell types in the dermis. The dermis contains connective tissue, sebaceous glands, muscle fibres, nerve plexuses and never fibres, sweat glands and blood vessels. The effects of high doses on blood vessels are visible as erythema and later as haemorrhages, which may appear as small (peteachiae) or larger (purpura) lesions. The peak onset of purpura occurs 3-4 weeks after irradiation, and can be produced by doses of 4-6 Gy. Following high doses of radiation to the dermis, a second wave of erythema is produced as a result of damage to the deep dermal plexus of blood vessels.

Temporary epiliation may result after a single brief exposure to 3-5 Gy of low-LET radiation and is most severe 2-3 weeks after irradiation. Permanent epilation may occur after a single exposure to more than 7 Gy, or to 50-60 Gy fractionated over a period of weeks Hair on the scalp is more sensitive than the beard or body hair.

Skin on the anterior aspect of the neck, antecubital and popliteal areas is most sensitive to radiation, followed by that on the anerior surfaces of extremities, the chest and abdomen. Thereafter, skin on the face (not strongly pigmented), the back and posterior surfaces of extremities, the face (strongly pigmented), the nape of the neck and the scalp are of decreeing sensitivity. Skin on the palms and soles is least desensitize to radiation.

The long-term effects of radiation on the skin, which develop months or years after exposure, include changes in pigmentation; atrohy of the epidermis, sweat glands, sebaceous glands and hair follicles; fibrosis of the dermis; and increased susceptibility of trauma and chronic ulceration. These changes result in part from depletion of fibroblasts and in part from injury to blood vessels in the dermis. It is possible that the loss of epidermal cells may also contribute.

The Reproductive System

The germ cells of the ovary and testis are very radiosensitive and their irradiation impairs fertility in both sexes in a dose-dependent manner. In male spermatozoa are continuously produced in the seminiferous tubules of the tests. Spermatogonial stem cells divide to produce primary specrmatocytes, which, in turn, give rise to secondary spermatocytes, spermatids and mature spermatozoa. In humans the development of mature sperm from spermatogonial stem cells takes about 10 weeks.

Spermatogonial stem cells are more radiosensitive than are postpermatogonial cells stages. The second and third stages of spermatogenesis, from preleptotene spermatocytes through to thc spermatids, are not affected by doses of less than 3 Gy. After such doses, postsprmatogonial cells mature and a normal sperm count can be maintained for approximately 46 days. the time-period required for the development of spermatozoa from prepleptotene spermatocytes. Thereafter, the sperm count will drop, approaching azoospermia by 10 weeks following a dose in excess of 1 Gy. Sterility will remain until the surviving 'stem' spermatogonia are able to repopulate the semiferous tubules in humans a dose of 2.5 Gy may cause temporary sterility for 1-2 years, while a dose of 6 Gy will often cause permanent sterility. The threshold dose for permanent sterility does not increase appreaciablyon fortification of irradiation over days or even weeks.

The mature oocyte is the most radiosensitive germ cell stage in females. Exposure of both ovaries to an acute dose of more than 0.65-1.5 Gy can cause temporary sterility. With doses below 2-3 Gy, enough immature occytes may survive to restore fertility. It has been estimated that the ovary can withstand 6-20 Gy or low-LET radiation in highly fractionated or protracted exposure regimes. The threshold dose for permanent sterility decreases with age, probably owing to decrease in oocyte number with age.

An important consideration in germ cell irradiation is the potential increase in mutation incidence in the offspring. In general, irradiation of the female is less damaging than irradiation of the male in regard to the induction of mutations. This is due to greater lethal radiosentivity of mature oocytes, thereby decreasing the number of viable cells carrying mutations which could be passed to the offspring.

The genetic consequences of a given dose can be reduced if a time-interval is allowed between irradiation and conception. This is due to the variation of radiation of sensitivity with stage of germ cell development. In malses irradiation immediately prior to conception, so that mature sperm are irradiated, increases the sensitivity to mutation induction. This is a direct consequence of the greater resistance of mature sperm cells to the lethal effects of radiation. If the time-interval between irradiation and conception is longer, so that the sperm involved in fertilization are irradiated during an earlier developmental stage, then fewer mutations result,.

The Digestive System

Radiation damage to the epithelia cells of the mucous membranes in the moth and throat evokes inflammation and swelling, with ulceration and necrosis developing after high doses. Mucosal injury is greatest in the cheeks, soft palate and hypoglosal region, and less in the gums, hard palate, nose, posterior wall of the throat, tongue and larynx. Following doses of up to 10 Gy of low-LET radiation, the mucosal surfaces recover after 2-3 weeks. With doses of 10-20 Gy extensive mucosal necrosis occurs after 4-5 days and recovery is much slower (1.5-2 months).

The salivary glands are radiosensitive but may recover even after high doses provided that the dose in given in a fractionated regimen. Following 50-70 Gy of conventionally fractioned X-rays, the salivary glands undergo necrosis, atrophy and fibrosis, which results in reduced salivary flow (Rubin and Casarett, 1968). In humans there may be a loss of taste after doses as low as 2.4-4.0 Gy (Congar, 1973).

The glandular mucosa of the stomach, small intestine and colon respond more rapidly and tolerate less radiation in a single exposure than do the squamous cell mucosa of the oral cavity, pharynx, oesophagus and anus. Radiation damage to the germinal epithelium in the mucosa interferes with cell renewal and may cause ulceration and, possibly, denudation of the affected mucosae. Exposure of a large part of the intestine to an acute dose in excess of 10 Gy may lead to the induction of the rapidly fatal gastrointestinal syndrome, as described earlier. With regard to long-term effects, fibrosis, stricture, intestinal perforation and fistula formation may develop months of years after exposures as complications arising from radiation injury to he gastrointestinal tract.

Of the paenchymtous organs of the digestive tract, the liver appears to have the lowest threshold for injury. Impaired liver function results from exposure of the whole organ to 30 Gy of conventionally fractionated therapeutic X-radiation. Changes which may include damage to centrilobular veins, with thrombosis and portal hypertension, may lead to hepatic failure ascites and death. With partial irradiation of the liver, substantially larger doses can be tolerated.

The Respiratory System

The respiratory system can tolerate considerable localized radiation injury, as, for example, when a small part of lung is heavily irradiated for therapeutic purposes. If, however, both lungs or a large proportion of lung tissue is irradiated with doses of greater than about 8 Gy, a fatal pneumonistis may develop after a latent period of 1-3 months. The earliest signs of radiation injury to the lungs are oedema and changes in blood circulation, which precede pneumonitis.

Individuals who survive the acute inflammatory phase of pneumonistis may later develop pulmonary fibrosis and core pulmonale. With a wholebody dose of more than 8 Gy, bone marrow failure may occur before severe lung damage becomes evident. The target cell population responsible for pneumonitis after irradiation is unknown, but type-II alvelopar cells are implicated and vascular injury may be contributory.

In the case of the upper respiratory tract, including tissues of the nasopharynx, larynx, trachea and bronchi, doses in excess of 30 Gy in 2 Gy fractions are required to cause ulceration atrophy and fibrosis (van den Brenk, 1971).

The Nervous System

Radiation-induced damage to the spinal cord, including demyelination and delayed necrosis of neurons in the white matter and damage to the fine vasculature, my develop between 6 months and 2 years after exposure (Rubin and Casarett, 1968). Typical neurological symptoms resulting from this damage include numbness, tingling, anaesthesia, paraesthesia, weakness and paralysis.

The brain is relatively resistant to radiation damage, with a dose of about 15 Gy required to produce deleterious effects. Necrosis of the brain, associated with demyelination and damage to cerebral vasculature, may occur within 1-3 years of receiving a dose of 55 Gy delivered over about 5½ weeks to the whole brain, or about 65 Gy delivered over 6½ weeks to a small part of the brain. This may lead to neurological symptoms and, in some cases, death. Many months after accidental or therapeutic irradiation in range over. 10 Gy, leukoencephalohathy, electroencephalographic changes and functional disturbances have been reported in humans, especially children. In addition, detectable morphological and physiological changes in children have been reported following a dose of 1-6 Gy (Ron *et al.,* 1982). With regard to the peripheral nervous system, damage may occur at doses above 60 Gy delivered in conventional fractionated radiotherapy regimens (Rubin and Casarett, 1968).

The Cardiovascular System

The heart is not a particularly radiosensitive organ, but a dose of 40 Gy, in conventionally fractionated radiotherapy, may cause myocardial degeneration, while a dose of more than 60 Gy to the entire heart may lead to death from pericardial effusion or constrictive pericarditis. If only a part to the heart is irradiated, tolerance is greater, but degenerative changes and fibrosis in exposed tissues may occur following a dose of 60 Gy.

A dose of 40-60 Gy will cause changes in the blood vessels in all organs (Rubin and Casarett, 1968). Vascular permeability and blood flow will increase in the early phases of the response. Endothelial cell degeneration, thickening of the basement membranes and progressive sclerosis will follow within a few months. Blood vessels may undergo late changes, including focal endothelial proliferation, thickening of the wall, narrowing of the lumen and decrease in blood flow. It has been suggested that vascular damage may play a major role in most forms of late radiation-induced tissue injury (Law, 1981).

The Endocrine System

Endocrine glands, including the thyroid, parathyroid, adrenal and pituitary glands, have a low cell turn over rate in normal adults, and are therefore relatively radioresistent, if, however, these glands are in growing or proliferative state, they will be more radiosensitive.

In children irradiation of the tryroid gland by external gamma-radiation or internally desposited radiodine can lead to hytpthyroidism and growth retardation (Conard *et al.,* 1975). In adults thyroid damage with myxoedema has been reported to develop between 4 months and 3 years after fractionated X-ray therapy with doses of between 26 and 48 Gy for tumours in the neck.

The pituitary and adrenal glands are less radiosensitive than the thyroid; in adults threshold doses of conventionally fractionated irradiation of about 45 and 60 Gy, respectively, are required to depress permanently the functioning of these glands. The threshold for severe functional damage following irradiation of the entire adult thyroid gland is approximately 25-30 Gy fractionated over 30 days; at lower doses subclinical damage may occur.

Although the female breast is relatively radiorestant during adult life, normal breast development may be impaired of doses of more than 10 Gy of conventionally fractionated X-irritation Gy of conventionally fractionated X-irritation are administered before puberty.

The Urinary Tract

Of the organs of the urinary tract, the kidneys are most radiosensitive, followed by the bladder and the ureters. The threshold dose for a fatal nephritis-like reaction in the kidneys, which can develop 6-12 months after irradiation, is estimated to be about 23 Gy of X-rays delivered in fractions of about 1 Gy over a 5 week period.

Radiation-induced, renal injury involves degeneration changes in the fine vasculature of the kidney and the epithelium of the nephron itself. Histologically, degeneration and depopulation of the renal tubules can be detected in the kidney within 6-12 months after irradiation following doses of more than 10 Gy; with high doses depopulation may be permanent, with degenerative changes in the vasculature. If the individual survives for several years after irradiation, the kidneys shrink in size, the capsule thickens and adheres to the cortex, and there will be cortical thinning and disorganization.

The bladder is less radiosensitive than the kidneys. With high doses complications, including cystitis, ulceration, fistula, fibrosis, contraction and urinary obstruction, may occur.

The Musculoskeletal System

Muscle, bone and cartilage are relatively resistant to the direct cytocidal actions of radiation. With doses exceeding 20 Gy administered during childhood in covenantally fractionated therapy, scoliosis, kryphosis, slipped upper femoral epiphysis and exostoses may be observed.

Early radiation damage in mature bone and cartilage is difficult to detect because of the paucity of cells, the abundance of matric, the radioresistance of the matrix and the mature cells, and the normally slow turnover rate or most of the matrix. The principal factor in radiation damage to these tissues is the injury to the fine vasculature supplying these structures. The degeneration and loss of dependent cells is secondary to interference with the blood supply, with changes in the matrix secondary to either of these changes. In the event of a large degree of vascular and cellular damage where there is degeneration and loss of many of the bone or cartilage cells, this will eventually be reflected in changes in the matrix, with development of 'radiation osteitis' or 'radiation chrondritis'. Whether or not the devitalized bone or cartilage results in structural disintegration depends on the degree at which occlusion of fine vasculature and loss of parenchymal cells occurs, and on the occurrence of complicating factors such as infection or trauma.

In a proliferative state, as, for example, in growing children, or during the healing of fractures, cartilage and bone may exhibit a greater response to radiation than when in the mature state. In children a dose of 1 Gy may cause some growth retardation, depending on the age tat irradiation and exposure conditions. With doses exceeding 20 Gy, administered in conventionally fractionated radiotherapy in childhood, skeletal changes, including scoliosis, kyphosis, slipped upper femoral epiphysis and exostosis, may occur. In adults, mature cartilage will tolerate 10 Gy fractio-nated over 4 weeks or over 70 Gy fractionated over 10-12 weeks; mature bone will tolerate up to 65 Gy fractionated over 6-8 week (Parker, 1972). Although these doses may be tolerated by adult bone and cartilage without necrosis, these tissues may exhibit increased susceptibility to trauma in the long term.

Large radiation doses (500 Gy) are required to cause necrosis of muscle which involves disruption of the fine vasculature and microcirculation, with increased capillary permeability, oedema and inflammation. At lower doses the acute oedematous and inflammatory response to vascular damage is more moderate and transient. However, the associated vascular damage and connective tissue reactions from acute interstitial oedema and inflammation may progress to cause delayed secondary degeneration, atrophy, or necrosis and fibrosis of irradiated muscles.

Stochastic Effects

The acute or early effects of radiation as described above result mainly from cell killing. By contrast, some late effects of irradiation result from damage to surviving cells which is transmitted to their progeny. Damage to germ cells may results in a genetic mutation that is expressed in a later generation; in the case of somatic cells, the result may be cancer induction in the exposed individual. Cancer and the induction of hereditary damage represent the stochastic effects of irradiation and regarded as the principal risks to health from low doses of radiation.

Radiation Carcinogenesis

Radiation is effective both as a carcinogen and in the treatment of cancer. The use of radiation in cancer therapy is based on its cell-killing ability, when administered in sufficiently large dose to replicating malignant cells. For cancer induction sublethal doses of radiation are important.

Several general principles apply to the induction of tumours by radiation. As a carcinogen, radiation is unique in that it can cause cancer in almost every tissue of the body, and radiogenic cancers are indistinguishable from those cancers which arise naturally or as a results of other carcinogens. Leukaemia (except for chronic lymphatic leukaemia) is the most frequently induced cancer. Chronic lymphatic leukaemia, squamous cell carcinoma of the cervix and Hodgkin's lymphoma are not induced by radiation.

Prior to the appearance of an induced tumour there is a latency period, the length of which depends on the type of tumour, its growth rate and metastatic form. The latency period for leukaemia is 2-5 years, while for other tumours

10 or more years is usual. There is also a delay before the initially 'transformed' cell or cells begin to divide to form a tumour, and there may be a further delay before the tumour assumes the 'malignant' characteristics of growth and spread. Radiation carcinogenesis is thought to be a multistage process involving initiation, promotion and progression.

Various factors influence the probability that an individual exposed to radiation will develop cancer. Current information suggests that sex has little or no effect on radiation carcinogenesis, while increasing age is associated with a decrease in radiation-induced tumours. Irradiation conditions, including the dose delivered, the time-period over which the dose is received and the radiation quality, are also important. Genetic constitution may be influential. Others factors, such as the host's susceptibility, living habits and exposure to other toxic agents, may contribute to cancer development.

Population exposed to moderate to high levels of radiation form the basis of radiation risk assessment and are fundamental to the development of models of radiation carcinogenesis in man. The most useful human data on the risk of radiation-induced cancer in terms of the length of time of follow-up and population size have been obtained from follow-up studies of the incidence of tumours in survivors of the Japanese atomic bombings at Hiroshima and Nagasaki during World War II, and from medically irradiated populations. Occupationally exposed individuals, e.g. certain groups of workers in the nuclear industry, also represent a potentially useful source of data, although as yet they yielded little quantitative data on cancer risk estimates.

The Life Span Study of the Japanese atomic bomb survivors represents the largest single study population examined for age and sex trends with a wide range of doses and currently has a follow-up period of over 45 years. Of about 280,000 individuals who survived the bombings, 80,000 have been followed up, with about 24,000 deaths,

5000 of which were caused by cancer; some of these were in excess of the number expected and have therefore been attributed to radiation. For those survivors exposed as adults, almost the entire course of induced cancer is now known; however, for those exposed as children the picture is still incomplete.

Investigations of medically irradiated population contributing useful information on the risk of radiation-induced cancer include the follow-up of over 14,000 ankylosing spondylitic patients given a single course of X-rays to ameliorate pain associated with disease, follow-up studies of patients irradiated as part of their treatment for cervical cancer or benign breast disease and follow-up of children irradiated for an enlarged thymus or for tinea capitus (scalp ringworm). In the ankylosing spondylitic patients, it has been shown that the relative risk for all neoplasms, other than leukaemia or colon cancer, more than 25 years their first treatment, is lower than that in the earlier years (5-24.9 years after treatment). This is in contrast to the results of follow-up studies of the Japanese atomic bomb survivors and of patients irradiated as part of their treatment for cervical cancer. In both instances the relative risk for all neoplasms (other than leukaemia and colon cancer) increased with time since exposure.

As yet no study population has been followed up for a long enough period to yield the lifetime incidence of cancers following irradiation. The overall risk for an exposed population must therefore be extrapolated over time, using models based on limited data. Two such projection models are used; an additive risk model and a relative risk model. The additive or absolute model postulates that the annual excess risk arises after a period of latency and then remains constant. In this case the risk from radiation appears to be additional to the natural incidence. The relative or multiplicative risk model postulates that the distribution of excess risk follows the same pattern as the time distribution of natural cancers—i.e. the excess is given by a constant factor applied to the age-dependent incidence of natural cancers in the population. Because the natural incidence of cancer; increases with increasing age, this model predicts a large number of radiation-induced cancers in old age. While it is to possible to distinguish between the two models for most cancers, for leukaemia and bone cancer (which have shorter latency periods) it has been established that these fit the absolute risk model.

Most of the data relating to human radiation carcinogenesis are derived from exposures at high doses and dose rates from which it is impossible to deduce the shape of the dose-response relationship, especially at low doses. Frequently the data are fitted to linear and linear-quadratic relationships. The former assumes that the excess cancer incidence is proportional to dose; the latter implies that at low doses cancer incidence is proportional to dose squared. In extrapolating the risk of cancer from high to low doses, the linear model implies that the risk per rad is the same at high and at low doses, the linear-quadratic model implies a smaller risk per rad at low doses. Because risk estimate are associated with a large degree of uncertainty, and are dependent on the choice of model used to extrapolate from high to low doses, they should not be viewed as definitive, but as the best available estimates based on inadequate data. Despite the difficulties associated with estimating the risk of radiation-induced cancer, the number of fatal malignancies induced cancer, the number of fatal malignancies induced by sparsely ionizing radiation in the range of 1 Gy is reported to be the order of 10^{-2} per sievert (UNSCEAR, 1988).

Dose-response relationships for radiation-induced cancers vary, depending on the tumour type and the radiation quality. For low-LET radiations, the incidence of many types of cancer increases with increasing dose, up to a maximum which usually occurs in the dose region 3 and 10 Gy. Thereafter, the cancer incidence decreases with increasing dose. The shape of the dose–response curve is the result of two phenomena: a dose-related increase in the proportion of normal cells transformed into a malignant state, and a dose-related decease in the probability that such cells may survive the radiation exposure. Both phenomena normally operate but to different degrees, depending on the dose and tumour type. The decreasing slope at high doses is attributed to the killing of the radiation-initiated cells from which tumours eventually arise. For densely ionizing neutron irradiation, tumour induction in animals in general, follows an almost linear curve at the lower end of the dose scale and exhibits little dose-rate dependence. For X- and gamma-rays the dose-response relationships tend to be curvilinear and concave at low doses. Tumour induction is dose-rate dependent, in that a reduction in the dose rate, of fractionation of the dose, reduces the tukour yield.

Hereditary Effects

Radiation-induced hereditary effects may be dominant or recessive, appearing in the first or later generations, respectively, and may involve changes to single gene or to the gross structure of a chromosome. A gene mutation involves a change in the structure of DNA and may involve the base composition, the sequence, or both. Chromosomal changes can involve the loss or addition of a chromosome, chromosome breakage and translocation.

Radiation-induced nutations represent an increase in the frequency of the same mutations that already occur spontaneously or naturally within a species. Since radiation-induced mutations are indistinguishable from those which occur naturally, large sample sizes are necessary to detect nay increase in their frequency caused by radiation. Human data relating to the genetic effects of radiation are scarce, with the exception of the follow-up of survivors of the atomic bombings of Hiroshima and Nagasaki (Neel et al., 1989). Estimation of genetic risk from radiation in humans is therefore based predominantly on animal data. It should be noted, however, that the result of *in vitro* studies of human cells, in conjunction with the limited evidence from

Hiroshima and Nagasaki, suggest that humans are not especially sensitive to the induction of chromosome aberrations and gene mutations by radiation (Neel *et al.*, 1989). Genetic risk is estimated on the basis that the doses received are genetically significant—i.e. that they are received by individuals before or during the reproductive period.

In using the data from animal studies to make quantitative estimates of genetic risks in man, three important assumption are made unless there is evidence to the contrary:

(1) The amount of genetic damage induced by a given type of radiation under a given set of conditions is the same in human germ cells and in those of the test species used as the model.

(2) The biological factors (e.g., sex, germ cell stage and age) and physical factors (e.g. radiation quality and dose rate) affect the magnitude of the damage in similar ways and to similar extends in humans and in the experimental species from which extrapolations are made.

(3) At low doses at low dose rates of low-LET irradiation, there is a linear relationship between dose and the frequency of genetic effects.

The genetics risks from radiation can be estimated by either the direct method or the doubling dose method. The direct method estimates the incidence of genetic diseases resulting from mutations or chromosomal disorders as a function of dose, and ignores the natural rate of these diseases in a population. By contrast, the doubling dose method involves a comparison between the rate of radiation-induced genetic disorders and the spontaneous incidence of these diseases in the population, and is expressed in terms of the dose required to double the spontaneous incidence of gene or chromosomal disorders.

On the basis of animal experiments, which have shown an approximately linear increase in point-mutations with radiation doses of 1-100 mGy, it is assumed that the increased irradiation of humans will result in a proportional increase in mutation frequency (Searle, 1989). Point-mutation frequencies of between 1 and 10 per million cells per Gy for human lymphoblasts (Grossovsky and Little, 1985; Konig and Kiefer, 1988), and less than 20 mutations per million cells per Gy for erythroblasts in A-bomb survivors (Langlois et al., 1987), have reported.

Survivors of the A-bombs have been studied for four genetic indicators: (1) abnormal outcome of pregnancy (stillbirth, major congenital defects, or death during the first postnatal week); (2) childhood mortality; (3) sex chromosome abnormalities; (4) mutations resulting in electophoretic variation in blood proteins (Schull et al., 1981). For these four parameters, differences between the children or proximally and distally exposed survivors were in the direction expected if a genetic effect did result from irradiation. However, none of the findings was statistically significant.

On the basis of mouse data (Russell and Russell, 1956; Russell, 1965), the doubling dose for low-rate exposure in humans was estimated by the Biological Effects of Ionizing Radiation (BEIR) II Committee of the US National Academy of Sciences to be in the range of 0.5-2.5 Sv.

Preconceptual Irradiation and Cancer Induction

There is considerable experimental evidence of the induction of genetic abnormalities by preconceptual irradiation of either parent. Searle (1989, and references therein) has estimated that the risk factors for a mutation at a specific locus in F_1 mice after paternal irradiation is about 0.001 per cent per Gy. From data such as these, UNSEAR (1988) has estimated that the total genetic risk for all loci in F_1 and F_2 humans after parental irradiation is about 0.3 per cent. This is in line with risk estimates for general congenital malformations in the offspring of irradiated male mice (0.5 per cent per Gy) (Kirk and Lyon, 1984; Nomura, 1982).

Interest in the induction of cancer-proneness by proconceptual irradiation has been stimulated recently by the results of a reanalysis of the incidence of leukaemia in children living near the nuclear installation at Sellafield in the UK. Gardner et al. (1990) reported that the incidence appeared to be associated with paternal employment at the plant and the recorded doses of radiation received by the fathers during the periods of their employment. It was suggested that these doses, although low, may have increased the risk of leukaemia in the offspring. The implication of the hypothesis is that if the association is truly causal, then it would follow that the risk of cancer arising from irradiation of pre or postmemeiotic germ cells must be very high.

The risk factors calculated from the data of Gardner et al., (1990) depend upon the period of preconceptual assumed to be important. These would be in the range of about 2 per cent per Gy for a lifetime dose to about 20 per cent for a 6 month dose. The problem arises in that risk factors of these magnitudes are vastly in excess of those normally expected for mutation at defined loci, as determined in radiation genetic studies in the laboratory. There are some experimental data, however, that are supportive. Nomura et al., have reported the induction of lung tumours and leukaemia after paternal irradiation in three strains of mice. The risk factors were found to be dose-dependent and varied with mouse strain, the germ cell stage at the time of irradiation and the type of tumour induced. Some responses in the offspring were also noted for preconceptual irradiation of female mice. The risk factors of a few per cent per Gy found in some of the studies imply that, in these experimental systems, induced mutations leading to cancer induction occur at much higher frequencies than those normally found for other types of mutations arising from preconceptual irradiation.

Effects of Parental Irradiation

Development harm to an individual exposed to radiation in utero is not easily classified as a stochastic or a non-stochastic effect. Irradiation of the developing embryo and foetus may result in death, malformation or growth retardation. The observed effect is dependent on the radiation dose, the dose rate and the gestational stage at which irradiation occurs. Prenatal irradiation effects are due to the fact that foetal tissues are continuously differentiating and growing, and fetal development follows a predetermined pathway; irradiation of the developing organism with the subsequent killing of embryonic or foetal cells at critical developmental stages can cause disruption in the normal complex sequence of events.

Gestation may be divided into three major stages: preimplantation, which extends from fertilization until the embryo attaches to the uterine wall; organises, which represents the period during which the major organs are developed; and the fetal stage, during which growth of the preformed structures occurs. The relative duration of each of these periods, the length of intrauterine life, and the state of differentiation or maturation of any one structure, with respect to maturation of any one structure, with respect to the others, varies between different animal species.

The preimplantation period is most sensitive to the lethal effects of radiation. Irradiation at this stage does not result in growth retardation, and few if any abnormalities are produced. If the irradiated preimplantation embryo survives, it will continue to grow and develop normally. At the preimplantation stage the embryo consists of a small cluster of cells, so that, if a few cells are killed by radiation, one or two cell divisions will rectify the damage. If, however, a larger number of cells are killed, the embryo will die and become resorbed.

Irradiation, during Organosis can induce cogenital defects. In the mouse a dose of 2 Gy during the period of maximum sensitivity can produce 100 per cent malformations in the offspring at birth (Russell and Russell, 1954), although in man radiation-induced malformations of structures other than the central nervous system are uncommon. This is probably related to the fact that the sensitive period for the induction of congenital malformations during organosis in humans represents a smaller fraction of the total period of gestation compared with that in small rodents. In humans, however, CNS development is occurring for much of gestational period, which makes it is likely target for radiation-induced damage. Consequently, the principal effects of irradiation during the period of organosis in humans are microcephaly and mental retardation.

Embryos exposed to radiation in early Organosis exhibit the most severe intrauterine growth retardation, from which there may be recovery later (i.e. temporary growth retardation). Irradiation in the foetal period lead to the greatest degree of permanent growth retardation.

Irradiation during the foetal period, which extends from about 14 days onward in the mouse, and 6 weeks onwards in man, can result in damage to the haematopoietic system, liver, kidney and developing gonads, the latter affecting fertility. Higher radiation doses are required to cause lethality during the foetal stage that at earlier developmental stages. In man the most commonly reported effects of *in utero* irradiation are microcephaly, mental retardation and other central nervous system defects, and growth retardation. Other effects including spina bifida, deformities, alopecia of the scalp, divergent squint and blindness at birth, are also recognized (Murphy and Goldstein, 1930).

Follow-up studies of individuals exposed *in utero* during the atomic bombings of Hiroshima and Nagasaki have shown that microcephaly can result from an air dose (Kerma) of 0.1-0.19 Gy. In addition, an increased incidence of severe mental retardation has been reported in the A-bomb survivors exposed in utero (Otake and Schull, 1984). A child was classified as severely mentally retarded when he/she was 'unable to perform simple calculations, to make simple conversation, to care for her/himself, or he/she was completely unmanageable or has been institutionalized'. The probability of radiation-related severe mental retardation is essentially zero with exposure before 8 weeks after conception, is maximum with irradiation between 8 and 15 weeks, and differences between 16 and 25 weeks. After 25 weeks and for doses below 1 Gy, no case of severe mental retardation has been reported. On the assumption that the induction of the effect is linear with dose, the probability of induction per unit dose was estimated at 0.4 and 0.1 per Gy at 8-15 and 16-25 weeks after conception, respectively (Otake and Schull, 1994). The period of highest risk of severe mental retardation coincides with the period of most rapid proliferation of neuronal elements, and with the migration of neuroblast cells from the proliferative zones to the cerebral cortex. It is thought that severe mental retardation results from radiation interfering with this normal sequence of events.

Prenatal irradiation with diagnostic X-rays has also been associated with the subsequent development of leukaemia and other childhood malignancies. In the Oxford Childhood Cancer study, irradiated children received between 1 and 5 films, with a dose of 0.2-0.46 rad per film. While these studies have been interpreted as indicating that relatively low doses of radiation results in an increased incidence of cancer during the first 10-15 years of life, by a factor of 1.5-2.0, they do not prove that in utero irradiation caused the malignancies. It has been suggested that the irradiated mothers represent a select group whose children are more prone to cancer and that the irradiation is coincidental. The strongest evidence in support of a causal relationship between irradiation and childhood cancer is that provided by Mole (1974) in an analysis of the Oxford data relating to twins. Twins who were X-rayed more frequently than singletons were found to have a higher incidence of childhood cancer.

11

Toxicology and Disasters

Introduction

Disasters (great or sudden misfortunes: *Concise Oxford Dictionary,* 1990), occur from time to time. Because they are portrayed and analysed extensively in the news media and subjected to careful examination in subsequent public enquiries, they become entrenched in everyone's mind. Unfortunately, the ideas on how to handle or prevent potential disaster situations occurring have often been developed from the lessons learnt from analysing previous disasters. In many cases disasters can be avoided and effects of accident minimized by careful planning. In addition, by examining how to handle the consequences of an accident once it has occurred, it should be possible to mitigate the effects. It is these thoughts that have led to legislation aimed at considering the safety aspects of certain hazardous situations at an early stage in order to minimize the likelihood of their becoming disasters.

Some disasters are the consequence of a toxicant entering a biological system and creating a damaging perubation to that system. These effects may be largely environmental (e.g. the consequences of an oil tanker spill in coastal water) or they may affect human health, either directly (through ingestion of contaminated drinking water or inhalation of a toxicant as it is dispersed in air) or indirectly (e.g. via uptake, etc., into food species). Thus, a knowledge of the effects of toxicants can be important when examining disasters and potential disaster situations.

In this chapter involved in planning to prevent disasters occurring are discussed first. This is followed by an evaluation of different types of disasters or serious incident involving toxicants. Although purely environmental effects should not be ignored, the examples chosen are all associates with human health effects. Afterwards approaches to the planning associated with preventing disasters due to toxicants and mitigating their effects are discussed.

Theoretical Considerations

Many of the concepts used in analysing major hazards and minimizing their potential for causing disasters have their origin in engineering concepts associated with the design of military equipment, aircraft and nuclear plant. As a consequence, the definitions used need examining, especially as difficulties can ensue if toxicologists and chemical engineers employ different intepretations of the same words. Although 'hazard' and 'risk' are interchangeable terms to the general public, they have separate meanings in the context of risk assessment, so their definitions will be examined carefully.

Hazard

Hazard is an intrinsic property of a substance or situation. The Royal Society Study Group on Risk Assessment (1983) defined hazard as 'the intrinsic situation that in particular circumstances could lead to harm'. The Institution of Chemical Engineers Working Party Report (1985) used the words 'a physical situations with a potential for human injury, damage to property, damage to the environment or some combination of these' and went on to define a chemical hazard as 'a hazard involving chemicals or processes which may release its potential through agencies such as fire, explosion, toxic or corrosive effects'.

Because the latter definition was intended for the process industries, it did not include potential radiation effects from nuclear plant failures. Such potential effects are also hazards (Health and Safety Executive, 1988a).

A toxicological definition to hazard called it 'the qualitative nature of the adverse, effect resulting from a particular toxic chemical, physical effect or inappropriate action'. This toxicological definition used carcinogenesis and asphyxiation as examples of toxic hazards. Thus, it is compatible with the engineering definitions.

A major industrial hazard is 'any man-made hazard which has the potential to cause large-scale injury and loss of life from a single brief event' (Health and Safety Executive, 1988a). Major industrial hazards include nuclear power stations as well as chemical process plant, and the definition of a major chemical hazard as 'an imprecise term for a large-scale chemical hazard' by the Institution of Chemical Engineers (1985) is entirely compatible. In circumstances where plant failure is to the cause of a disaster, the initiating event may be prolonged; thus, a major hazard can be any naturally occurring or man-made hazard can be any naturally occurring or man-made hazard that has the potential to cause large-scale injury and loss of life from a single event. For chemicals or radiation to represent toxic hazards, they must be present in sufficient quantities to exert toxic effects on the individual. If they are to be major hazards, must be present in quantities which, if released or dispersed, could result in effects being seen in many people.

Risk

Risk differs from hazard, as it involves a consideration of the probability or likelihood of a consequence occurring as well as what the consequence might be. The Royal Society study group (1983) defined risk as 'the probability that a particular adverse event occurs during a stated period of time or results from a particular challenge'. The Institution of Chemical Engineers (1985) extended the statement of 'the likelihood of a specific undesired effect occurring within a specified time or in specified circumstances'. The go to say that it may be either a frequency (the number of events occurring in unit time) or a probability (the probability of a specific event following a prior event), depending on circumstances'. If risk is quantified, it is statistically based parameter.

The Relationship Between Hazard and Risk

In engineering terms for toxic risks the individual risk is obtained by identifying possible events resulting in hazardous releases and by analysing potential failure mechanisms which would allow the release in order to determine their likely frequency and size (Health and Safety Executive , 1989a). The hazard is a quantitative statement of the potential consequences of release. Central to this approach is the assu-mption that events occurring during ordinary use do not constitute a significant risk. Societal risk is expressed numerically as the frequency (F) that there will be a disaster harming more than a particular number (N) of people, and can be aggregated in the form of an F-N curve. Lees (1980), Marshall (1987) and Health and Safety Executive (1989a,b) give more detailed discussion of these ideas.

Toxicological risk has been called ' the probability that some adverse effect (e.g. cancer) will result from a given exposure to a chemical' (Hodgson et al., 1988). When human data are available, they are the actual or estimated frequency of occurrence of an event in a population. However, the toxicological risk is often based on extrapolation of information from animal studies. These studies indicate that the substance is hazardous to the animal and therefore that there is a (presumed substantial until otherwise proven) probability that the hazard may also occur in man.

For the purposes of analysing the potential health effects that could arise from a major hazard, the effects are considered as 'hazard to man' and the difficulties in extrapolating information to man are part of the uncertainty in defining the hazard.

Individual and Societal Risk

There are two principal types of risk which can arise from major hazards: individual risk and societal risk. The Health and Safety Executive (1988a) has called the individual risk associated with major industrial hazards 'the risk of any particular individual, either a worker or a member of the public.' A member of the public is considered to be 'either anybody living within a defined radius from the establishment or somebody following a particular pattern of lie'. Societal risk was 'the risk of society as a whole, as measured, for example, of a large accident causing a defined number of deaths and injuries'. Although the individual risk is remains the same for each persons, the societal risk if governed also by the number of people likely to be affected. The individual risk of living 1 km for major hazard (industrial or natural) remains the same irrespective of whether the hazard is located in an unpopulated area or in a city, but the societal risk is very different!

Risk Assessment and Risk Management

The concepts of hazard and risk are fundamental to analysing the causes of disasters and to preventing their recurrence. However, these concepts must be contained within a framework of analysis and management if they are to be applied usefully to a given situation. In practice there is a multistage process involved in handling any hazard, and most of the people analysing and managing hazards from industrial plants have engineering or chemistry backgrounds. Their specialism cover plant design and failure rates, event and fault tree analyses, dispersion modelling for releases of clouds of substances and rates of combustion, etc., for explosions and burning gases (Lees, 1980; Withers, 1988). Geologists are often the principal interested in the causes of natural disasters involving toxicants. There are 'overt' disasters where a clear point source can be identified readily. Only when the substance released is a toxicant or is transformed into a toxicant will any toxicological input become important. This input will largely in defining the hazard; it will be concerned with identifying whether the agents present are toxic and defining the combination of exposure size and duration likely to produce a given toxic effect. Clinical toxicologists are also able to advise on the treatment of victims following an incident, i.e., they can have a role in the event of an incident occurring.

'Diseminated' disasters are those which only become apparent because of evidence of effect. Identifying the cause when the effect is ill-health may require persistent, painstaking research. If the suspected cause is non-infective, the investigation team will need the assistance of toxicologists in identifying the agent responsible.

Often risk can be managed in more than one way. The aim of risk management is to reduce the risk, both in terms of the frequency of an event and in terms of the nature of the potential consequences to an acceptable or tolerable level. This involves choices as to what chemical and physical agents are usable by society and in what circumstances. It involves selecting which processes to employ when manufacturing, using or disposing of these agents and their waste products. It also involves choices on where to site plants (in the case of man-made hazards) and methods of waste disposal, and whether to permit housing, etc., developments around major hazards. It is also concerned with examining how to handle the consequences of an untoward event at a particular site (emergency planning). What is an acceptable, or at least a tolerable, risk is a separate, but interlined problem, which depends on a number of factors. Some of these factors are listed in Table 18.1. Ultimately, government decides whether a societally regulated risk is generally tolerable. Individuals or groups of individuals may attempt to vary the decision as it relates to their specific circumstances and perceptions. In the final analysis risk acceptability revolves around political and personal decisions, although it is to be hoped that such decisions are based on scientific data.

Serious Incidents Involving Toxicants

Many disasters are the results of major hazards fulfilling their potential for harm. They are part of a continuous spectrum of possible consequences which can arise from a point hazard. These consequences range from minor difficulties through serious incidents until, in the worst cases, they become disasters. Most of these disasters are not due to toxicants. Their primary effects are physical in nature, and include crush injuries and burns. Other disasters may be due to failure to meet adequate standards associated with ordinary exposures to potential toxicants. This failure may be because the appropriate knowledge was not available and the standard, in consequence, inadequate. Alternatively, it may be because of some accidental or international deviation from the standard. A classification of disasters is given in Table 18.2. This classification is based on the type of event which caused the disaster or serious incident.

Health effects due to toxicants may result from inhalating or from absorption through the skin or gastrointestinal tract. Inhaled toxicants may be gases, liquids (aerosol mists) or solids (dusts, fumes). Particle size is important when particulate material is inhaled, since, if inhaled, a particle may be deposited the lung alveoli or, as a result of the 'trachea-bronchial escalator' it may be swallowed. An inhaled toxicant may cause injury to lung, it may restrict the transfer of oxygen (asphysiation), or it may act systemically in a particular organ (including skin). Skin and eye effects are often phenomena of surface contamination.

Gastrointestinal absorption may contribute to the overall toxicity of inhaled material. However, it is the main route of entry for those toxicants which are transmitted to man in food or water supplies.

Natural Disasters

Disasters due to natural causes include phenomena caused by the movement of the earth's crust as well as the consequences of abnormal weather. In general, these types of disasters cause injuries due to physical effects or disease due to infective organisms. Toxicants are rarely involved, and then usually secondarily, except in the cases of volcanoes and gas emission from lakes. Asphyxiation can be caused by emitted gases and irritant dusts, as well as respiratory dysfunction, bronchial obstruction and pulmonary oedema.

Volcanoes

Volcanic eruptions can be divided into two types—explosive and effusive. Each type may present different health hazards. In volcanic eruption, magma (molten rock and associated dissolved gas below the earth's surface) is extruded to the surface. When it reaches the surface, it may appear as liquid (lavae), fragments (pyroclastic debris) and exsolved gases. In effusive eruptions these flows are usually slow-moving, as releases are steady and most of the limited amount of dust produced is non-desirable. Explosive eruptions tend to be more dangerous, the principal toxic hazards being to ash release and gas emission. Volcanoes may change their nature from one type to the other.

The gas emitted by volcanoes is principally steam, but ıncludes carbon dioxide, carbon monoxide, hydrogen sulphide, sulphur dioxide, hydrogen chloride and hydrogen. Plumes normally disperse by dilution in the atmosphere and are carried on the wind above human settlement. However, sulphur dioxide, hydrogen chloride or hydrogen fluoride may occasionally be present in sufficient quantities to contaminate air within settlements quantities to contaminate air within settlements, water supplies and animal feedstuffs. Denser-than-air gases, principally carbon dioxide and hydrogen sulphide, can flow into valleys and low-lying basins and displace oxygen, giving rise to asphyxiation. A *nuee ardente* (a cinder cloud carrying trapped gases can flow rapidly down slopes and many also endanger life.

Pyroclastic debris (tephra) and ash products vary in size. Blocks and bombs are large (over 64 mm), lapilli vary between 2 mm and 64 mm, and cinders, and ashes are smaller particles, Lapilli and ash, when released to the atmosphere, rise in a hot convention club which may be transmitted widely (several hundred kilometres) downwind. Eventually they fail to earth and blanket large areas. Finer particles are deposited further away. The particles have the ability to cause darkness during daylight hours. Ash products include respirable particles containing significant levels of crystalline silica (quartz and cristobolite). Volcanic ash can affect the respiratory track and eyes. Severe tracheal injury, pulmonary oedema and bronchial obstruction can occur, leading to death from pulmonary injury or suffocation. Ash may also act as a respiratory tract and eye irritant. Irritation and inflammation of the upper and lower respiratory tract may persist if low-level chronic exposure occurs.

Lava is molten rock, the liquid product from the volcano. It is derived from the molten magma, but differs from it because the dissolved gases in the magma escape with the reduction of pressure which occur as the material approaches the surface.

Debris flows occur when loose rock mixes with surface water or groundwater and flows as a mass of rock, mud and water.

This description of volcanoes is inevitably very short and much simplified. More detailed information can be found in Sheets and Grayson (1979) and Newhall and Fruchter (1986).

Vesuvius, Italy, AD 79

Perhaps one of the best-known historic volcanic eruptions is that of Vesuvius in Italy in AD 79. A contemporary description of the eruption and its effects on one victim is provided by Pliny the Younger in two 'letters' to Tacitus (Radice, 1969). More detailed information on the eruption and its consequences has been obtained during archaeological investigation of the sites at Pompeii and Herculaneum, both of which were buried in the eruption (Jashemski, 1979; Sigurdsson *et al.*, 1985).

Vesuvius has been quiescent for many centuries before the eruption of AD 79. The first sign of its reawaking was an earthquake in AD 62 which damaged almost all the buildings in Pompeii. Then came the eruption of AD 79. There were three phases of this eruption. The first stage was expulsion of the vent plug on 24 August. This was followed by expulsion of ashes. There were six surges and pyroclastic flows during the ash eruption.

Both Plinys were at Misenum when Vesuvius erupted, together with Piliny the Elder's sister (Pliny the Younger's mother). Pliny the Elder who was in command of the Roman fleet at Misenum, gave instructions that a ship would be made ready so that he could investigate the phenomenon. However, by the time the ship got under way, with the elder Pliny, he changed the mission to one of attempting to rescue the people living along the shore of the bay at the foot of Vesuvius. Pompeii and Herculaneum were probably being buried at this time, the former from disposition of lapilli and ashes and the latter from a mud and tephra flow. Pliny found his mission impossible because of the falling debris near the shore, and eventually made port at Stabiae, where he stayed the night. During the night the courtyard of the house in which he was staying filled with ashes and debris. On the morning of 25 August it was still dark at Stabiae after dawn. Pliny the Elder went to the shore to investigate the possibility of escape by sea, and died. Pliny the Younger described the death as because 'the dense fumes, choked his breathing by blocking his windpipe which was constitutionally weak and narrow and often inflamed'. In modern terms this might be described as asphyxiation.

The crew of the ship later successfully got away, and the young Pliny and his mother were evaluated from Misenum on 25 August as ashes started falling there. Both survived. Although the 'letters' only describe ash and lapilli, there was also a lava flow on the north side of the volcano. The results of excavations at pompeii suggest that at least 2000 people died. Most deaths were probably due to asphyxiation caused by inhaling the hot ash material in the first surge of the ash eruption, but some might have been due to thermal shock (Sigurdsson *et al.,* 1985). Presumably many more deaths went unrecorded.

Mount St. Helens USA. 1980

A much more recent volcanic eruption was that of Mount St. Helens, in the Cascade range in the west of North America. Premonitory earthquakes started on 20 March and, towards the end of April, a bulge developed in an area to the north of the summit (Buist and Bernstein, 1986). On 18 May a major earthquake occurred, the roof of the bulge slid down hill and an explosive blast took place. Large quantities of ash, superhearted stream and gas were released. There were five additional explosions over the following 5 months and ash falls accompanied four of these eruptions.

There were 35 known deaths and at least 23 people missing without trace following the eruption (Baxter *et al.,* 1981, 1983; Buist and Bernstein, 1986). Asphyxiation was the cause of death in 18 of the 23 victims autopsied. Ash probably acted as an irritant to the respiratory tract and eye, causing tracheal injury, pulmonary oedema and bronchial obstruction in those dying. The irritation of the respiratory tract continued as the results of chronic low-level exposure to ash, but there appeared to be few long-term sequelae. However, any potential pneumoconiotic effects from the single massive exposure to silica could not be detected within the short time-span since the eruption. Interview studies of patients with pre-existing chronic lung disease showed that the ash fall exacerbated the conditions in these patients. There were dose-reared increase in the prevalence of three psychiatric syndromes associated with disaster stress—namely generalized anxiety, major depression and post-traumatic stress. The duration of effect was related to the level of disaster stress suffered by the subject.

The toxic effects seen in the victims of the Mount St. Helens eruption were largely those due to the nature of the ash deposited. Fortunately, the toxic gases that were emitted were vented to the atmosphere and diluted to non-toxic levels through dispersion.

Other Natural Disasters

Volcanoes are not the only natural phenomena which can cause major disasters due to toxic substances. On 21 August 1986 there was a catastrophic release of gas from Lake Nyos, Cameroon. The cloud of gas was lethal at distances up to 10 km from the source. About 1700 people, 3000 cattle and many other animals dies, mostly from asphyxiation. An earlier, smaller release from Lake Monoun, also in Cameroon had resulted in 37 deaths, presumably from similar causes.

The generally accepted cause of the disaster is that , because of the geochemical and geophysical characteristics of the Cameroon rocks and the geological conditions in the Lake Nyos area, waters rich in carbon dioxide develop. The gas accumulated in the lake of near-saturating conditions. Although the trigger mechanism for the release is unknown, a small disturbance would have been sufficient to cause degassing in the form of a large release of the carbon dioxide. The gas cloud produced was denser than air and dispersed through the river valleys. Simultaneously, a water surge resulted in the loss of about 200,000 t of water from the lake. The release was heard as a series of rumbling sounds lasting 15-20 s, and one observer reported seeing a white cloud rise from the lake.

Many people lost consciousness rapidly and survivors woke 6-36 h after the event, weak and confuses. Cutaneous erythema and bullae were present in about 19 per cent of survivors treated in hospital. Very limited pathological investigations on those dying suggested that carbons dioxide was the toxicant, as it appeared that the potential toxicant, as it appeared that the potential toxicants, carbons monoxide, cyanide or hydrogen suplhide, were not relevant to the cause of death. Reports of the odour of sulphur compounds were probably a result of the sensory hallucination due to exposure to high levels of carbon dioxide.

This disaster was a consequence of the special geology of the area. Therefore, although a rare event, it does illustrate that natural disasters involving toxicants are not confined to volcanic releases.

Man-made Disasters

Plant Failure

Plant failure are a well-known cause of major disasters. Those involving the release of toxic chemicals or radioactivity are relevant to toxicologists and some examples are examined here. A much more comprehensives collection of cases studies of the causes and consequences of chemical plant failure in major disasters, written from the chemical engineer/risk assessor' point of view, is given in Marshall (1987.

Seveso, Italy, 1976

An escape of toxic substances occurred at an industrial plant at Seveso, Italy, in 1976. The circumstances surrounding the escape and the potential health effects caused by the escape were investigated by Parliamentary Commission of Enquiry (Orsini, 1977), and both the engineering and chemical aspects of the incident have been reviewed recently (Marshell, 1987; Skene *et al.,* 1989). The incident was important because of its influence on European Community legislation (the 'Sevesco' Directive) concerned with major industrial chemical hazards.

The plant produced trichlorophenol by reacting tetrachlorobenzene with sodium hydroxide. Following the reaction, the solvent (ethylene glycol-xylene) was partially vacuumdistilled off by the end of shift, at which time the heating and agitation were switched off. Some 7.5 h later safety plate on the reactor vessel burst and there was a consequent venting of the reaction mixture, including approximately 2-3 kg of the impurity dioxing (2,3,7, 8-tetracholorodibenzo-p-dioxin) to the atmosphere. Once in the atmosphere the dioxin was spread over a wide area downwind of the plant and settled on fields and houses.

Three major zones were identified according to the levels of dioxins present in the vegetation and soil. The resident population in the zones were 733, 4800 and 22, 000 people, respectively, in the most contaminated, middle and last contaminated areas. A medical surveillance programme was undertaken on these people.

Apart from burns arising directly from contact with the caustic reaction products, the other major effect was chlorance. This was reported some 6 weeks after the accident, with a frequency correlating approximately to the levels of dioxin in the soil. By the end of 1978 the chlorance had disappeared.

Repeated-dose animal studies suggested that dioxin could cause porphyriaed and was hepatotoxic. In animal studies on reproductive effects, dioxin was a potent fetotoxin and teratogen. Hepatocarcinogenicity has also been established in animal studies. Thus, these effects were examined in the follow-up to the single acute exposure at Seveso.

Studies on liver effects, including porphyria, in 700 children failed to identify significant illness, although two indicators of liver dysfunction, gamma-glutamyl transferase and alanine amino-transferase, were slightly elevated in boys from the most contaminated zone.

A birth defects register was set up after the disaster. There were not birth defects that could be unequivocally linked to dioxin exposure among the limited number of births to residents of the high-exposure zone. In addition, although there were wide variations in the spontaneous abortion rate between zones, these could not be ascribed to dioxin. Examination of chromosomes in aborted tissue following artificially induced abortions suggested that there might have been a higher frequency of chromosomal aberrations in fetuses from mothers potentially exposed to dioxins, but it was not possible to establish where these aberrations would have led to adverse reproductive outcomes.

Perhaps the greatest long-term worry from the Seveso incident was cancer. All those exposed have now been followed up for 10 years (Bertazzi *et al.*, 1989). There are no excesses of overall mortality or mortality due to all cancers. Risks of deaths from certain individual cancers and from cardiovascular disease were elevated, but they could not be related to exposure patterns. Although restricted by the short observation time and the small numbers of deaths from certain, causes, they study seems to suggest that there have not been the feared large increases in the overall numbers of deaths from cancer.

The Seveso incident illustrates how an accidental release of a chemical may be perceived by the general public as a major disaster. So far, few, if any, human deaths have resulted from the single-dose exposure to dioxin. Those suffering chlorance or burns recovered. Fears of large numbers of people being affected by potential long-term effects have not been confirmed despite scientific study. Nevertheless, the Seveso incident is important, as it raised the general awareness of the potential that there may be for ill-health following major plant failure.

Bhopal, India, 1984

Methyl isocynate was a stoxic substance responsible for a major disaster at Bhopal, India, in December 1984 at factory manufacturing the pesticide carbaryl.

The cause of the accident was the introduction of water into a storage tank containing methyl isocyanate. This resulted in the production of carbon dioxide :

$$CH_3NCO + H_2O \rightarrow CH_2NH_2 + CO_2$$

The combination of rising temperature due to a run away exothermic reaction coupled with gas evolution led to a build up of pressure which caused 30-35 t of methyl isocyanate to be vented to the atmosphere in a 2-3 h period (Marshall, 1987). The venting occurred during the night and the cloud dispersed over a densely populated area.

Estimates of the number of deaths which resulted from the release vary between 1700 and 5000, with up to 60 000 people being seriously injured. Survivors reported that the vapour cloud gave off considerable heat and had a pungent odour. Irritation, coughing and choking were early symptom, and were followed by vomiting, defecation and urination, and panic, depression, agination, apathy and convulsion. Although severe eye effects, including temporary blindness, were seen in many survivors, they did not persist. Initial lung effects (oedema, focal atelectasis) were probable caused of death and led, in survivors, to more persistent changes inflammation. Serial studies showed that some survivors improved, that there was no change in some and that some wrosened. Liver and kidney function appeared to be normal in survivors.

The Bhopal incident illustrates man be important points. First, although the reasons for the war entering the methyl isocyanate tank were never clearly identified, the consequences were made substantially worse than they need have been because several of the design safety features had been rendered unusable and because there were substantial numbers of shanty houses right up to the factory fence. Also, there was a paucity of toxicological data on methyl isocyanate prior to the incident, which has now been rectified by undertaking substantial studies in animals as well as following up the victims (Bucher, 1987). At the time of the incident there was only one substantial published report on the toxicity of methyl isocyanate, and that was restricted tos an animal study on the acute effects following single exposure.

Chernobyl, USSR, 1986

Chernobyl, 80 km north of Kiew, USSR (now Ukraine) was the site if probably the worst accident to have occurred at a nuclear plant.

In April 1986 a test was being conducted on a reactor during shut-down for routine maintenance. However, the planning of the test was poor and safety devices were deliberately switched off to allow the test to proceed. By the time it was realized that something was wrong, uranium oxide fuel elements in the upper part of the core had probably started to disintegrate because of the high temperatures. Explosions followed which released considerable quantities of radioactivity to the atmosphere, much of which was dispersed over the Soviet Union and western and northern Europe.

By 1 year after the event only 31 people had died as a result of it. They died in the immediate aftermath of the accident, from acute radiation sickness. However, there could be a total of over 10,000 premature deaths due to cancers caused by the radioactivity, of which 35 might be in the UK, over the following 50 years (Henderson, 1987). This has to be set against the approximately 7 million anticipated deaths due to cancers in the UK over the same time.

The radioactivity from the accident was washed from the skies and entered food chains, notably in areas of high rainfall. In the UK this led to the banning of the sale for human consumption of sheep meat from badly affected areas for over a year. Subsequent to the accident, the people in the area around Chernobyl were evacuated. They have not been allowed to return and the area is being converted to a national park where human activity, including farming, is banned. This disaster is one in which future illness and premature deaths are the primary effects on man. It is this fear of the future effects of radiation which has made the nuclear industry so heavily regulate in comparison with other industries.

Fire

Thermal injuries, heat stress and physical trauma from collapsing structures are obvious problems in major fires. However, fire statistics indicate that deaths consequent on being overcome by smoke are the most common type of death (Committee on Fire Toxicology, 1986). Such deaths and incapacitation are due to the evolution of toxic combustion products. As toxicant are likely to be funnelled upwards and diluted to non-toxic levels in unconfined fires, major fire disasters usually occur in confined spaces when it is not possible to escape from the effects of the toxic combustion products.

Smoke includes all airborne products from the pyrolysis and combustion of materials (Committee on Fire Toxicology, 1986). Full oxidation of susbstances present in fires would result in such products as carbon dioxide, water (steam), nitrogen dioxide, sulphur dioxide and chlorine. However, complete combustion rarely occurs and other products such as carbon monoxide, soot (particles), hydrogen cyanide, hydrogen chloride, hydrogen fluoride, acrolein and other organic materials are often present. The toxicity of fires therefore arises from the evolution of smoke (including gases, dust/fume and aerosol), containing irritants and asphysiants and, potentially, carcinogens. Those most at risk will normally be the firefighters in close proximity to the fire, and thus near enough to inhale undispersed toxic smoke and gases.

Potentially, risks from acute health effects of dispersed combustion products may occur in warehouse fires such as that at Brightside, Sheffield (Health and Safety Executive, 1985). Onlookers who were in close proximity to the fire may have acquired sore throats and chest symptoms due to effects from the fire. However, potential combustion product toxicants were dispersed to levels thought too dilute to pose a risk to the general population within very short distances. Asbestos roofing materials were dispersed widely in this fire, but the longer-term health effects for people exposed to single doses of dispersed fire products were considered to be minimal.

Two examples of disasters in which the evolution of toxic combustion products from fires contributed significantly are given below. In both examples most of those who died were incapacitated by the effects of inhaling toxic smoke and gases in relatively confined spaces, and thus became unable it move to less polluted atmospheres.

Manchester Airport Crash, UK, 1985

One area where there is a potential for disasters due to toxic is aircraft fires. An example of such a catastrophe was the Manchester Airport crash of 1985 (Air Accidents

Investigation Branch, Department of Transport, 1989).

On 22 August 1985 a British Airtours Boeing 737 aircraft bound for Corfu was taking off from Manchester International Airport when the left engine suffered an uncontained failure which punctured a wing fuel tank access panel. The leaking fuel ignited and burnt as a large plume of fire trailing directly behind the engine. The crew abandoned take-off and cleared the runway by turning onto a taxiway as they stopped. A light wind carried the fire onto and around the rear fuseleg. After the aircraft stopped, the hull was penetrated rapidly, and smoke and possibly flame entered through one of the cabin laft-doors which had just been opened. Fire subsequently developed inside the cabin and generated a dense black toxic-irritant smoke. Despite prompt attendance by the airport fire services, the aircraft was destroyed and 55 people (53 passengers, 2 crew) died, one after 6 days in hospital. All those who died on board the aircraft had general congestion and oedema of the lungs with carbon particles in the air passages, consistent with inhalation of smoke. The cause of death was inhalation of smoke for 48 people and direct thermal injury (burns) for only 6 passenger.

Of those engulfed by smoke, only 38 (47 per cent) survived. The survivors reported that a single breath of the cabin atmosphere was burning and painful, immediately causing choking. They experienced drowsiness and disorientation. Eight survivors actually collapsed, but recovered sufficiently to get out from the plane. Most of the deaths due to inacapacitation might have been prevented if the people concerned had been protected from smoke or if external assistance had been more quickly available. All except one of the survivors of the immediate accident made their exit within 7 min of the aircraft stopping. The only passenger recovered alive by firemen as taken out after 33 min; he died 6 days later from severe pulmonary damage and associated pneumonia.

The thermal decomposition products of cabin materials included toxic irritant gases, such as carbon monoxide, hydrogen chloride and hydrogen cyanide. Some fluorinated materials (used as decorative films) yielded hydrogen fluoride. It was probably the combined effects of toxic combustion products which caused death. Elevated levels of carbon monoxide and cyanide and the metabolic product of cyanide, thiocyanate, were found in all except six of those dying on board the plane. Individually lethal levels of carbon monoxide were found in 13, and of cyanide in 21 of these people (9 had leaves of both substances, either of which could have been lethal); for the remainder, the sum effects from the total amounts of toxic materials present probably caused death.

This aircraft accident is an example of a disaster where many of those who died might, in other circumstances, have been rescuable. One element that played a part in the disaster wds disablement by the smoke from a fire in a confined space before exit from the space could be achieved. This has encouraged investigations into the potential for placing smoke-hoods of suitable design on aircraft for passenger use in this type of emergency. Investigations into possible 'in-cabin' firefightiog systems in order to slow down the development of toxic atmospheres were also undertaken as a consequence of this disaster.

Kings Cross (London) Underground Station, UK, 1987

Thirty-one people died an many more were injured in an escalator fire at Kings Cross Underground station. The fire took place in the evening at an extremely busy Underground station where four lines cross. Access to the three deep lines (Piccadilly, Victoria and Northern) is from the ticket hall below the main line station forecourt. The ticket hall is approached by subways from Kings Cross and S. Pancreas main line stations and from street level. According to the Inquiry Report (Fennel, 1988), the fire started in the Piccadilly line escalator, among an accumulation of grease and detritus (but, fibre and debris) on the running tracks, possibly as a result of a lighted match passing through the skirting board. This fine preheated the balustrades and decking, which were wooden. As a consequence of a 'trench' effect, the fire initially burnt cleanly and then produced dense, black smoke. 'Flashover' occurred as the fire erupted into the ticket hall. The deaths all occurred among people in the ticket hall at around the time 'flashover' occurred.

The Inquiry did not pursue in detail the question of cause of death for the 31 people who died, but concluded that many deaths were due to the toxic effects of the smoke rather than to burns. In the report the Inspector says:

> 'After hearing expert evidence about the role of toxic gases in the fire and the findings of pathologists on post-morton tests, I determined that the cause of death in individual cases could not be pursued any further in this Investigation. On the evidence available to me reliable assessment could be made of the relative importance of various materials present in the station to the production of toxic fire fumes or to the sources of toxic materials found in the bodies. Although separate statutory Coroner's Inquests were held, the Coroner decided not to take the matter further.'

A major part of the inquiry focused on the procedures by which London Underground dealt with escalator fires. It was clear that the Underground lacked an adequate approach to safety in terms of their attitudes to safety matters, their attention to staff training in safety and their equipment and procedures to be used in emergencies. The lack of preparedness led to an emergency becoming a disaster.

Food and Drink

Mass poisonings due to contamination of food or drink may be considered disasters. Many episodes of this type of mass poisoning are the consequences of bacterial or fungal contamination of food consumed by the victims. If the causative agent is pathogenic, then health can suffer. However, a portion of such poisoning is due to the introduction of a chemical toxicant into the consumed material, either directly or via a food chain.

Because of the indirect way in which the contamination affects man, it can be difficult to demonstrate cause and effect. Ill-health may occur indirectly, in a species (man) remote from that (e.g. wheat) to which the toxicants was administered, possibly after transmission through a food chain (fed to farm animals, etc.) or directly (in bread). It may be some time before the toxicant accumulates sufficiently for the victim to exhibit symptoms of ill-health, or for the ill-health to be manifest following ingestion. Consequently, considerable detective work may be needed in order to identify the cause of ill-health, and on occasion it may never by properly characterized.

A series of examples of incidents involving contamination of food or water follow. Further examples can be found in Aldridge (1987).

Adulteration of Food or Drink

Adulteration (debasing by adding other or inferior substances: *Concise Oxford Dictionary,* 1990), of foodstuffs and deliberate poisoning by admixture in food have gone on from time immemorial. Adulteration for commercial reasons was rife in the eighteenth and nineteenth centuries (see Smullen, 1989). Bread from bakers often contained chalk, lime, lead salts or even bone to make it look white. Leaves of hawthorn, sloe or ash were used to dilute tea. With hindsight several of these adulterants were toxic chemicals and may have had disastrous consequences for the recipients. Deliberate adulteration, when it occurs, is still capable of causing major disasters.

Ginger Paralysis, Mid-west and South-west USA, 1930

During Prohibition in the United States, the Prohibition Bureau ruled that the USP 'fluid extract of ginger' was a non-potable beverage and its sale was not restricted. This beverage was an alcoholic extract of material from the ginger plant and was freely drunk. An adulterated 'fluid extract of ginger' entered circulation through dealers (non-pharmacists), mainly in Ohio and Tennessee early in 1930. Cases of paralysis started occurring in mid-February. Adult men were the principal victims and those showing symptoms seemed to do so some 10 days to 3 weeks after drinking the suspect ginger extract (Smith and Elvove, 1930). Ultimately some 50,000 people were affected (Morgan, 1982).

The paralysis appeared as soreness of the muscles of the arms and legs, with occasional numbness in the fingers and toes. Foot and wrist drop and weakness of the fingers developed. The symptoms were found in distal parts of the limbs and were more marked in the feet and legs. This neuropathy was primary axonopathy caused by demyelination and dying back from the distal end of the long nerves. In some cases recovery was very limited (Aldridge, 1987).

In a very detailed piece of work, the causative agents was identified chemically as tri-*ortho*-cresyl phosphate. Both the adulterated ginger extract and the presumed adulterant, tri-ortho-cresyl phosphate, were found to cause the symptoms of the neuropathy in calves, chickens and, to a much less marked degree, rabbits, but had little effect on monkeys or dogs following oral ingestion.

Toxic Oil Syndrom, Spain, 1981

Toxic oil syndrome was a previously unknown disease syndrome which appeared in Spain in May, 1981, Principally in Madrid and north west provinces (World Health Organization, 1984; Aldridge, 1985, 1987). The epidemic was at its peak in mid-June and faded away thereafter. By March 1983, 340 deaths had occurred and over 20,000 cases had been recorded.

The disease developed in two phases. In the acute phase, a pleuropneumonia sufficient to cause respiratory distress and death in severe cases as present. This pleuropneumonia did not respond to antibiotic treatment and about 20 per cent of survivors did not recover completely. A chronic phase of the disease, a sensorimotor peripheral neuropathy of variable appearance, developed, together with scleroderma-like skin changes. There was little evidence of central nervous system involvement.

Although initially thought to be due to an infective agent, the syndrome was rapidly associated with the consumption of an oil sold for food use in 5 litre cans by itinerant salesman. The oil was rapeseed oil, denatured with aniline, intended for industrial use. In most cases the oil had been refined, mixed with other seed oils, animals fats and poor-quality olive oil, or chlorophyll, but in the cases of a small number of victims in the Seville area (well away from the main outbreak) the re-refined oil had not been further processed. The unsolved problem in toxic oil syndrome is the exact nature of he (presumed) chemical toxicant. Despite considerable effort aimed at its identification, the precise toxicant has not been identified.

Accidental Contamination

As opposed to deliberate addition of materials to foodstuffs or drinks, accidental addition of toxicants can also occur. If the toxicant is sufficiently effective and affects a large number of people, a major disaster could result.

Pollution of Drinking-water in North Cornwall, UK, 1988

Mass intoxication in theory at least, could occur due to contamination of drinking-water supplies. That this is not such a remote possibility was demonstrated in 1988, when the South West Water Authority found that a truck load (20 t) of alum had accidentally been released into the drinking-water supply to Camelford, a small town in Cornwall, and the surrounding district, (Lowermoor Incident Health Advisory Group, 1989). The material was delivered into the treated water reservoir at Lowermoor Treatment Works. The pH of the water dropped below 5 and aluminium levels were raised to over 10mg l^{-1}, considerably above the 0.2 mg l^{-1} set on palatability grounds in the European Community Drinking Water Directive. Although initial advice from local sources suggested that little ill-health would occur, newspapers reported considerable acute health symptoms and speculated that there were potential long-term effects. The expert assessment was that the early symptoms of gastrointestinal disturbances, rashes and mouth ulcers were probably due to incident, but short-lived. Later complaints of joint and muscle pain, memory loss, hypersensitivity and gastrointestinal disorders may have been induced because of 'sustained anxiety naturally felt by many people'. The expert committee concluded that there was no adequate scientific foundation available for the speculation on potential long-term effects.

The incident is a sufficient reminder of the possibility of a disaster occurring as a result of contaminated water supplies. It also illustrates the difficulties which occur in allaying fears when the affected population receives initial advice which was, to quote the conclusions of the Advisory Group, 'contradictory, confusing and sometimes inappro-priate'.

Contamination of Food Storage–Epping Jaundice, UK, 1965

Epping Jaundice was an outbreak of jaundice which affected at least 84 people in the Epping area of London during February 1965. It was traced to ingestion of wholemeal bread made from flour contaminated with 4,4'-diaminophenylmethane. The chemical had spilled from a container on to the floor of a van which was carrying flour as well as chemicals.

In most of the cases jaundice and liver enlargement were preceded by severe, intermittent pains in the upper abdoment and lower chest areas of the body. Normally, these pains were of acute onset (50 patients), but sometimes onset was insidious (27 patients). Of the 57 patients further investigated, most has raised serum bilirubin alkaline phosphate and aspartate aminotransferees levels. Needle biopsies were performed on 4 patients within 3 weeks of the onset of symptoms; all showed considerable evidence of portal inflammation and the duct cholestasis and showed evidence of hepatocyte damage. The lesions was reproducible in mice given 4,4-diaminophenyl-methane (Schoental, 1968).

The patients slowly recovered over succeeding weeks.

The jaundice was the result of an accidental undected (until too late) contamination of a foodstuff because if was stored during delivery adjacent to chemicals which were insufficiently securely contained within the packaging. The chemicals were absorbed by the flour through the sacking and, following baking, were present in the bread.

Poisoning Due to Consumption of Foodstuff Not Intended for Human Consumption—Methylmercury Poisoning in Iraq, 1971-1972

An outbreak or organomercurial poisoning due to the consumption of treated gain by farmers and their families occurred in Iraq in 1971-72 (World Health Organization, 1976). There were 459 deaths and over 6000 furthers cases admitted to hospital.

Poisoning cases started to appear in hospitals in late December. Farming families only were affected and the cause of the poisoning was identified as consumption of home-made bread, an important element of their diet, made from wheat treated with seed dressing. There was a latent period of up to 60 days from first consumption to the appearance of signs and symptoms of poisoning, and in many cases consumptions of contaminated grain ceased before the symptoms occurred.

Symptoms included speech disturbances, abnormal behaviour, loss of auditory and visual acuity and ataxia. The severity. The severity varied from minimal effects to severe disability and death. Most of those showing only mild or moderate symptoms were symptom-free 2 years later, although symptoms were still present in severe cases. Mercury levels in hair were found to be good indicators of the dose of mercury received.

Organomercurials, such as the methylmercury involved in this episode, are fungicides, the methylmercury being used as a seed dressing to prevent wheat bunt and other crop diseases. Grain dressed with methylmercury was distributed to farmers between mid-September and early December, 1971. Although much of the wheat had been consumed before a cause-effect relationship had been established, surplus treated grain was withdrawn to storehouses once, the cause of the outbreak was known. The problem arose because wheat intended as seed for next year's crop was eaten by the farmers and their families rather than used for its intended function.

Environmental Pollution

The examples of major disasters arising from toxic substances so far discussed arise from contamination of the foodstuff. It is also possible for contamination to arise indirectly as a result of an environmental pollutant entering a food chain. Two examples of this occurred in Japan, at Minamata and Niigata.

Over the period 1951-1974 there were over 700 recognized cases and 80 deaths due to 'Minamata disease', and over 2000 other people had applied for recognition as Minamata disease patients. The principal geographical areas affected were in two prefectures, Kumamoto and Kagoshima, which border Minamata Bay. The disease occurred mainly in fishermen and their families who consumed large quantities locally caught fish containing high concentrations of mercury. The patients's nervous systems were affected with symptoms of sensory, motor and visual involvement. Domestic cats (presumably also largely fed fish) exhibited similar clinical signs, and abnormal behaviour occurred among crows in the affected areas. Cogenital effects also occurred.

The outbreak of poisoning at Niigata was first identified in 1965, with over 520 patients being identified by the end of 1974. The epidemic was also apparent in the domestic animal population.

In the Minamata outbreak the effects were due to organically bound mercury present in sludges from industrial plant. The mercury was used as a catalyst. Mercury from the sludge or from the waste-water outlet food chains and was bioconcentrated in both shellfish and fish. These were eventually consumed by man. At Niigata river fish from the lower reaches of the Agano river were the main foodstuff consumed which contained organic mercurial compounds. The source of the mercury was an industrial plant water-waste discharge containing low concentrations of mercury. Methylation took place in sediments and considerable bioconcentration occurred in the fish, as evidenced by the much higher levels of mercury in the fish when compared with the river water.

At both sites consumption of contaminated fish had gone on for a considerable time before the causes of the disease were identified. This points to the great difficulties involved in deriving a cause-effect relationship when the effect is remote from the source of the causative agent.

Although the particular examples chosen to illustrate this effect related to human health, other specises may be final consumer in a food chain. The story of the consequences of spraying persistent organochlorine insectisides, their bioconcentration in the food chain and their disastrous effects on raptor population because the concentrations reached were sufficient to cause eggshell thinning and failure to reproduce effectively, summarized in Smith (1986), is well known.

Interactions of Man and Nature

Mining

In genera, toxicants are unlikely to be a primary cause of a specific mining disaster, as the conditions causing ill-health are unlikely to develop suddenly. Historically, it is possible that disasters due to asphyxiation or the release of toxic gases occurred. Canaries were taken underground to act as fail-safe biological monitors for these effects. (When the singing ceased...) Nowadays forced ventilation makes these events extremely rare.

People have died as a result of lung cancer due to exposure to random in mines or of pneumoconiosis caused by exposure to coal dusts or silica, but the exposure to these agents was a consequence of inadequate working conditions rather than specific accidental exposures.

Waste Disposal

Inadequately thought-out disposal of wastes may cause major disasters.

Love Canal, USA

Love Canal was a waste disposal site which contained municipal and chemical waste disposed of over a period of 30 years up to 1953. Homes were built on the site during the 1960s. Leaching became a problem in the late 1960s, when chemical odours were detected basements. These were followed by fears of potential ill-health which led to considerably psycholgical stress. Dibenzofurans and dioxins were identified in the organic phases of leachates and were presumably derived from the disposal of waste products of the manufacture of chlorinated hydrocarbons. Animal studies, conducted on the organic phase of the leachate, indicated that there could be risks of immunotoxic, carcinogenic and tetraogenic effects (Silkworth *et al.*, 1984, 1986, 1989a,b). Low birthweights have been found in the offspring of resident of Love Canal (Vienna and Polan, 1984). Although follow-up was limited, no casual link has been established for exposure to chemicals and cancer in man (Janerich *et al.*, 1981). Nevertheless, serious social and psychological consequences have resulted from the use of the site for houses and the lack of understanding of the fears of residents initial apparent on the toxic properties of the chemicals dumped at the site (Holden, 1980).

Minimata and Niigata

The mercury poisoning at Minamata and Niigata, already described, were caused by the disposal of industrial wastes in such a manner that the toxicant was concentrated to dangerous levels in a food chain in the aqueous environment.

Conclusions

Toxicants, whether derived from nature or the chemical plant, can cause disasters. Identifying the cause is relatively easy when the toxicant is airborne and the ill-health occurs during or shortly after exposure. It is usually more difficult if the effects is mediated via the food or water supply and/or if the effect is not immediately apparent. The former have been called 'overt' disasters and the latter 'dilute disasters (Bertazzi, 1989). As 'dilute' implies some diminution of effect, it might be better to refer to the latter type of disaster as a 'disseminated' disaster.

In overt disasters due to airborne toxicants there is usually a primary event such as volcanic eruption or a plant failure. This is followed by dispersal of the toxicant, which depends on the buoyancy in air of the material released and the meteorological conditions at the time of release. Any immediate dose received by man will depend on the level and duration of the exposure. Only very sile post-event preventative measures can be used to minimize the dose received. Although usually ill-health is immediate, long-term effects such as carcinogenicity could occur. However, they are difficult to link to a primary event and are chiefly known for release of radioactivity. Toxic material can be deposited on to surfaces containment, to prevent ill-health due to continuing lower-level exposures, may be difficult.

Most known airborne toxicants involved major disasters affects the respiratory tract. Irrigatation, asphyxiation (chemically induced by binding of toxicant or physically induced by blockage of the respiratory tract) and pulmonary oedema are common. Cancers are frequent effects of radiation. Other toxic effects may occur in organs away from the respiratory system, although this appears to be rare. When airborne, the toxicant reaches the lung and respiratory system first; consequently they appear to the most frequently affected organ systems.

By comparison, 'disseminated' disasters are more difficult to identify and are often identified be effect. Tracing the cause may take a considerable time, particularly if the ill-health effect took some time to develop. Consequently it is more difficult to prevent exposures and it becomes more likely that a disaster will occur because of a voluntary oral intake of the food or water containing the toxic material. Organs other than the 'portal of entry' are more likely to be affected in such disasters, and withdrawal of the food, etc., causing the disaster may be too late to be an effective post-event preventative measure. In the absence of sufficient authoritative and accurate information, popular speculation generally favours the worst possible outcomes. However improbable. This is likely to worsen psychiatric consequence of the event and to complicate the emergency response. The provision of timely accurate advice in an understandable form is one need that must be considered when examining how to handle the consequences of a serious incident.

Approaches to Handling Major Hazards

One role of industry, individual governments and international organizations is to develop and implement procedures for preventing or minimizing the effects of potential or actual disasters. In most countries governments develop is series of legislative requirements in order to provide a framework of regulation within which to work. Rather than compare different national frame works, this section will concentrate on conceptual approaches to handling the risks arising from major hazards.

Assessment of potential hazards and assessment and management of the likely consequences are the key elements in any process for dealing with major hazards. In the case of toxic hazards, one aspect of the hazard evaluation is an examination of the likely toxicity of the materials involved in the potential disastrous situation, including prediction of the amounts of toxic materials likely to cause these effects. Procedures can then be adopted for the assessment of the risks associated with the various uses. Interacting with, and dependent on the risk assessment will be the approaches available by which the risks can be managed. These procedures of risk management differ fundamentally according to the type ('overy' or disseminated') of potential disaster envisaged.

Criteria for Judging Risk

'It is a risk?' Is usually questioned asked when a potential hazard is being examined. Once the concept of risk has been explained two questions will follow: 'what is the risk?' And 'is it acceptable/tolerable?'. This involves trying to define in general what is an acceptable or tolerable risk. Once acceptability (tolerability) has been defined, a method is needed in order to compare the risk for the particular problem under study with acceptable risk. That method may be qualitative, of the form 'acceptable'/'non-acceptable' based on a judgement of the data available against broadly defined criteria. However, for many purposes, including much risk assessment, many quantitative, numerical approaches are adopted. These numerical approaches are called quantified risk analysis. These quantitative analyses render decision-making easier, especially when choosing between options, as they give a clearer indication of the magnitude of a risk or of the relative risks for different options.

Criteria for judging the acceptability of a human health risk depend on three factors: the risk level (the frequency with which the event will occur); the definition of the biological event (death, serious injury, etc.); and the status of the receiving individual (a 'normal' or a 'vulnerable' individual).

Criteria against which to judge environmental effects are more difficult as the importance of a loss has to be considered as well as the size of the effect. Descriptions of damage levels constituting a major disaster are therefore judgements. One set of such end-effect criteria is that published by the UK Dept. of Environment (1991).

Risk Comparisons

When comparing risks, it is necessary to ensure that the particular hazard for which the risk is being calculated is the same for all the risks being examined, both in terms of the biological event and for the type of recipient. For many risks comparisons, that event is 'death' (in reality, foreshortening of life, often such that death occurs during or shortly after the event) as a result of an event and the individual responding is a 'normal person. Criteria for assessing this 'risk of death' have been obtained by comparisons with everyday risks associate with various activities. There are several level there is the 'trivial' 'negligible' or 'completely acceptable' risk. At the other extreme there is the 'intolerable' or 'unacceptable' risk. In between lies a range of risks which are tolerable under certain circumstances and/or provided they are minimized.

A risk of about 1 in 10^6 per year that the individual concerned will die from a given cause appears to be generally regarded in the United Kingdom as acceptable (Royal Society Study Group, 1983). This was justified by considering the death rates for different activities considered 'safe'. The risk of death for workers in recognized dangerous occupations is the order of 1 death per 10^3 per year; thus this is considered the highest bound to 'tolerable' risk for a lifetime risk. Any higher level is considered intolerable and unacceptable at all times. Because working in a 'risky' industry is, at least to some extent, voluntary, the individual risk just tolerable for a member of the general public living in the neighbourhood of a hazard is considered to be tenfold less (1 death per 10^4 per year). This approximately the risk from death in a road traffic accident and slightly less than the risk of developing any form of cancer. All of these risk criteria relate to individual risks and to average individuals.

A more conservative approach has been adopted in the Netherlands (Versteeg, 1988). It depends on the frequency of deaths from natural causes and is based on the idea that industrial activity should both increase the background mortality by more than 1 per cent. An upper bound of 10^6 deaths per year has been derived, with a lower bound of 10^8 per year being considered trivial.

In between the upper and lower bounds of acceptability lies a region where risks from known hazards should be reduced as far as reasonably practicable. This means that the cost of reducing the risk should not be disproportionate to the level of risk encountered. A small reduction in an already low risk may not be justified if it is very expensive.

Overt Disasters

Potential 'Overt' disasters can be averted or minimized by a combination of land-use planning and emergency planning. Good land-use planning can minimize the potential risks of a disaster by restricting the size of any interaction of event and consequence. A hazardous process of a large store of hazardous material can be sited well away from large numbers of people. Potential developments involving significant numbers of members of the public can be sited away from natural or man-made major hazards.

There will remain a residue of risk after appropriate land-use planning has been achieved. Occasionally there will be the situation where inappropriate combinations of people and major hazards occurred prior to the time when the need for appropriate land-use planning became apparent. In addition, other considerations, such as a need for local employment, may mean that other factors were decisive when the planning decision was made. The consequences, should the event occur, can still be substantially reduced, provided that appropriate emergency planning has been undertaken. This involves both enabling potential victims to survive better prior to treatment and making available appropriate treatment sufficiently rapidly.

Land-use Planning

Although the criterion of death can be employed in land-use planning, allowances need to be made for the uncertainties in developing this criterion for an individual within a population. Do we need the data for 5 per cent dying or 85 per cent dying? In addition, there may be serious, but sublethal, effects on health. These sublethal effects may be of great concern when handing toxic substances. In consequence, a broader concept, the 'dangerous dose', has been employed. The dangerous dose is a description of the exposure conditions producing a level of toxicity (Health and Safety Executive, 1989a; Turner and Fairhurst, 1989):

(1) Severe distress will be caused to almost everyone.

(2) A substantial fraction will require medical attention.

(3) Some people are seriously injured and require prolonged treatment.

(4) Any highly susceptible people may be killed.

This type of criterion reflects that there is a range of individual ill-health effects and imprecision in the level of overall effect seen in the population.

The type of population being considered may also differ according to circumstances. Rather than examining the frequency of achieving a given biological effecting terms of the event occurring in an average individual in a 'normal' population, it may be that the consequence should be considered for an individual from a population containing a large number of particularly vulnerable (or susceptible) individuals.

If the biological effect being looked at changes and the type of individual being examined is different, then the numerical value of any risk criterion ought also to be altered. When quoting a risk criterion for it, it is therefore necessary also to mention the effect and the type of recipient. Otherwise confusion reigns.

Some arbitrary ratios have been enunciated for the relationship between the risk criteria for exposure conditions, leading to 'death' and 'dangerous dose' in the same population (Health and Safety Executive, 1989a). The Health and Safety Executive has suggested that a risk of 1 in 10^6 per year for a 'dangerous dose' corresponds to a risk of 3.3 in 10^7 per year for risk of 'death'. Such a value will depend. In large measure, on the slope of the dose-response line; nevertheless, there is some evidence that might be considered to support the assumption. It can be calculated from a comparison of the relationship between classification on the basis of oral LD_{50} values based on the criteria in Health and Safety Executive, 1988c) and on the basis of 'evident toxicity' following an oral dose to young, healthy arts (van den Heuval *et al.,* 1987) that the ratio between these events which yields the same classification is approximately 4:1, As 'evident toxicity' is less severe effect than 'severe distress', a ratio of 3:3:1 is probably appropriate as a generalized, pragmatic assumption. Because risk is normally measured using logarithmic scales, this is a convenient value, as it represents a half-order of magnitude on such a scale.

A risk of criterion of 3.3 in 10^7 per year from when there is high proportion of 'highly susceptible' people receiving a 'dangerous dose ' has also been proposed in place of the 1 in 10^6 per year for a individual from population containing a normal balance of 'highly susceptible' individuals (Health and Safety Executive, 1989a). This is more aritrary. The identity of the 'highly suscepitable' people will depend on the effects seen, and this proportion will differ as effect differs. As homes for the elderly, caring institutions and long-stay hospitals are considered to contain a high proportion of 'highly susceptible' people, it would suggest that the occupants of such institutions are, in general, more susceptible to the effects of toxic chemicals. However, the choice of the ratio of 3:3:1 (again a half-order of magnitude) must be a pragmatic rather than a scientific decision.

Emergency Planning

Emergency planning is essentially concerned with handling the consequences after an event has occurred. It involves both immediate responses of emergency services and the medical management of the immediate and long-term health effects (Murray, 1990). Such planning is concerned with a much wider range of biological effects than death. These include 'severe health effect' (disability, requiring hospital treatment), and 'mild health effect' (discomfort or distress, detection or nuisance). ECETOC has defined three 'Emergency Exposure Indices', airborne concentration for exposures lasting up to a specified time, below which direct toxic effects are unlikely to lead to one of death/permanent incapacity, disability or discomfort.

Although hospital treatment may be essential for recovery from the severe health effects, it will usually have little influence in the case of the milder effects (discomfort).

There is also a need to plan for an appropriately sized event. One proposal categorizes three types of release: small but likely accidents, severe but reasonably foreseeable events and large unlikely events (Baxter *et al.,* 1989a). In the severe, reasonably foreseeable event is chosen for planning purposes, then it should be possible to scale up or down the response for an individual event relatively readily.

'Disseminated' Disasters

Essentially, 'disseminated' disasters should only occur as a result of failure of a regulatory mechanism resulting in exposure to a toxicant. That failure may be because a new effect was uncovered by the disaster. Alternatively, a known effect might have occurred because of non-adherence to pre-existing regulatory requirements. The primary means of control has to be preventative, ensuring that, under normal conditions of exposure the frequency of ill-health is acceptably low. A sufficiently rigorous enforcement system is also needed in order to ensure that failures in control which result in higher frequencies of ill-health to not occur. This type of approach is based on the conventional 'no effect' level and safety factors, leading to such concepts as maximum 'acceptable daily intake' and occupational exposure limits'. Where carcinogenic or other stockhastic risks are concerned, the approach will be to minimize exposure as far as is reasonably practical.

Determining Risk Levels

Determination of risk levels is required for overt hazards. There are essentially similar processes for determining risk levels for land-use planning and emergency planning (Health and Safety Executive, 1989a; ECETOC, 1991). The process can be divided into seven steps (Health and Safety Executive, 1989a).

(1) Identification of possible hazardous release events.

(2) Identification and analysis of the failure mechanisms which would allow a release to occur.
(3) Estimation of rates and durations of the release.
(4) Estimation of the frequencies of releases using the analysis of failure mechanisms.
(5) Estimation of the injury consequences of releases, taking account of mitigating factors.
(6) Combination of the frequencies and consequences to determine the overall risk levels.
(7) Judgement of the significance of the risk levels (by comparison with appropriate criteria).

Although this process was described for land-use planning in the vicinity of major industrial hazards in the UK, it can also be used more generally. Essentially, it can be described as three elements—a description of a source, a model for looking at the dispersion of the substance and a means of entering into the dispersion model parameters describing the conditions which will give a biological effect.

The source term for inputting into the dispersion model can be obtained by 'fault tree' analysis of the frequency of events (failure rates), by 'event tree analysis' leading to an estimate of failure rates or by engineering judgement based on historical event frequency. The actual method(s) chosen will depend on the type of release being studied and the available data. The sizes and durations of the postulated/actual release are also examined. For land-use planning there is a continuum of event frequency and size of release. Usually, sets of release sizes and durations are selected from the continuum and assigned appropriate frequencies. However, for emergency planning the process can be simplified by using the 'severe, but reasonably foreseeable event' as the appropriate basis on which to plan. This event was exempli-fied as a large hole in or fracture of a liquid chlorine pipe or of a road tanker delivery coupling at a chlorine installation. Scaling a response up or down should then be possible when an event actually occurs if the plan is sufficiently flexible.

The modelling then required is concerned with the

dispersion of the toxic cloud. Several models have been described. In general, these models require a knowledge of the buyont density of the cloud under different weather conditions. The dispersal conditions need to be combined with a function describing the combination of exposure concentration and time resulting in a defined effect. For example one concentration-time combination may be described as the 'dangerous dose' for land-use planning, while a different combination could be used for the outer boundary for 'discomfort' for emergency planning. When combined with the information on the source, the model is then used to calculate 'isopleths'. These are boundaries of areas within which, at a point time, the concentration-time combination of exposure to the toxic substance would exceed those expected to give the identified biological effect. An overall isopleth envelope can then be calculated for a given set of release conditions by combining the individual isopleths for each time point post-event.

The information on the various isopleth envelopes for different types of release and meteorological conditions, when combined using a knowledge of the frequencies with which these conditions occur, gives a generalized 'contour' for all source terms and dispersal conditions. This contour is a risk statement for individual risk for a person within the specified boundary. An estimate of societal risk can then be obtained if data on the distribution of people within the geographic area are inputted.

The Contribution of Toxicology to Hazard and Risk Assessment

The most likely direct hazards arising from a major accidental release of a toxic substance are the biological consequences of short-term exposure during dispersal of the toxicant. Longer-term or delayed effects should be considered as well as those more immediately apparent. Indirect consequences due to contamination of food or water supplies or to inhalation of dusts following settlement and subsequent disturbance are potentially important, but less immediate, problems, and should be amenable to post-event measures aimed at preventing significant exposure.

The Data Available

In theory at least, the ideal assessment of toxicity of a potential major hazard substance or agent would be based of accurate observations of the appropriate effect in man. Reliable reports on severe effects in man are, fortunately, few, and mainly as a result of accidental exposure or exposure in wartime. Controversy often surrounds the exposure levels associated with such studies. Results from studies on sublethal effects in man may be more plentiful. Nevertheless, the data on most substances are restricted to accidental exposures, often affecting only one or two people and rarely containing accurate exposure information. Except for radioactivity, human evidence concerning long-tear effects of single exposures to most agents and substances is virtually non-existent. Further studies which require deliberate exposure of men (or women) to dangerous levels of a substance or agent are unethical.

As a consequence of the limited human data, heavy reliance has to be placed on animal and other experiments in attempting to predict the adverse effects in the human population. Often these animal data are confined to short-term effects (sometimes only lethality) following single exposures. Prior to Bhopal, the information, available on the toxicity of methyl isocyanate was confined to a single published paper (Kimmerle and Eben, 1964) on short-term effects following acute exposure (Bucher, 1987). Also, many animal studies on the types of substances which might constitute major hazards were performed a long time ago and the data are by modern standards, of poor quality.

In view of the very variable nature of the toxicity information, it is essential to evaluate this information critically and to understand the uncertainties introduced as a consequence of the nature and quality of the data. This means that assessments will normally be conducted using the original reports or published papers.

As the information may be required for quantitative risk analysis, where possible it will need to be described in numerical terms. Uncertainty has to be handled by sensitivity analysis. By inputting various potential values for particular effects into the risk assessments, it is possible to discover the differences that variation of the input parameter will have in terms of the outcome, the areas of the map covered by the contour envelop related to a particular risk value. This sensitivity analysis is an essential part of the overall risk assessment.

Usually there are few, if any, data on the immunological, carcinogenic reproductive effects likely after single exposures to major hazard substances/agents. Indirect effects, mediated through food chain uptake and bioconcentration or disturbing settled material also need to be considered. If data are available, they should be evaluated. However, that evaluation will normally be descriptive as, except for the effects of radioactivity, there is currently no satisfactory way of obtaining the data in a form suitable for more quantitative approaches.

Problems of Extrapolation

The difficulties encountered in extrapolating from data in animals in evaluating the hazard to man, and hence, the risk, are similar, whatever, the nature of the hazard and rise being examined may be. The ways in which these extrapolations can be carried out have been described in great detail elsewhere. Three principal problems-intespecies variation, population heterogeneity (interindividual variation) and route-to-route extrapolation–are particularly relevant when data for major hazard substances are being examined.

Interspecies variation in biological effects is an important area of uncertainty in the evaluation. Toxicokinetic and toxicodynamic relationships between species, together with information on the relevant biochemical parameters in man, can lead to a better understanding of the relevance of results in a particular species for man.

Physiologically based toxicokinetic models for extrapolation between species have been developed in other areas of toxicology and are being used in the evaluation of the relevance of carcinogenic studies in animals for man. As many major hazard substances are lung toxicants, models based on the structure and function and on access of inspired area to the different part of the lung may also be important. As substances are taken into blood and more slowly exhaled, owing to the development of tissue reservoirs of the material, but nevertheless mediate their effect at the lung surface, the models for lung may need incorporation into toxicokinetic models. This type of modelling has not yet been applied to major hazard toxicants, probably because of a lack of suitable data. Nevertheless, it would help considerably in reducing the uncertainty of interspecies estrapolation. The models and the data are likely to be developed over the next few years.

In the absence of appropriate toxicokinetic models, extrapolation between species is more judgmental. Allometric scaling is an obvious technique to use. As both lung surface area (for absorption) and body weight or body surface area (for effect) can both be scaled allometrically, they are, in general, less applicable to inhalation studies when compared with studies using other routes of administration. The only possible approach often is to take the exposure effect data based on the most sensitive relevant species and check it against any relevant human data.

In addition to interspecies variation, it is necessary to consider interindividual variation and the nature of the population being studied. Animal experiments, particularly those performed in recent years, have been conducted using animals specially bread to limit variations in response, and are usually young, healthy individuals. In many older studies much less closely defined animals were used. The general human population is more heterogeneous still, containing groups of individuals who must be considered 'highly susceptible' because of age, genetic constitution or disease state. These interinidvidual variations are a factor which adds to the uncertainty when extrapolating from animal studies to effects in man or when extrapolating from a small sample to a large population.

Occasionally, toxicity data may be used which were obtained for a different route of exposure that for which they are being assessed (Pepelco and Withey, 1985; Pepelco, 1987). For example, in the absence of sufficient inhalation data it may be possible, in some circumstances, to make use of oral data and to relate them to equivalent inhalation exposures. However, comparisons cannot be made if there are substantial differences in toxicokinetic for the two routes. Often, effects on the lung are critical. These can be considered local effects, in which case it is not appropriate to extrapolate from oral data. Great caution is required when extrapolating data from studies suing different routes of exposure.

Modelling the Toxicity Information

The best way of relating exposure level, duration and effect for quantitative risk assessment is probably based on toxicokinetic and toxicodynamic modelling similar to that used for workplace exposure to inhaled gases and vapours. However, appropriate data are not available for most, if not all, major hazard substances, so other, more pragmatic, approaches are adopted.

A generally available pragmatic approach is based on the need to obtain: (1) a concentration-time relationship usually based on the mid-point (LC_{50} or EC_{50}) of the effect(s) being examined and (2) an appropriate set of exposure conditions that are taken to result in a particular level of effect in the population)(Turner and Fairhurst, 1989; ECETOC, 1991).

As the concentration-time (*c. t*) relationship often have to be based on LC_{50} or EC_{50} data for various times (they are frequently the only data available), they normally refer to mid-point concentration, that where the effect is seen in 50 per cent of the population. In general, the values have to be adjusted to yields boundary between effects (disability, with few immediate deaths for 'dangerous dose'; discomfort few disabled in the case of defining zones where people needing hospital treatment are likely to be located). The dose response may also need to be adjusted to account for differences in the make up of the population being examined. It make-up of the population being examined. It must be emphasized that any boundary will be approximate because of the nature of the data and the models being used.

In the early years of this century studies on the acute inhalation toxicity for a limited number of gases yielded mortality data suggesting the following relationship:

$$c.t = \text{constant}$$

(Habre, 1924). This is usually known as the Habre rule. More recent observations have suggested a more general relationship:

$$c^n.t = \text{constant}$$

(ten Berge *et al.*, 1985; Klimisch *et al.*, 1987; Marshall, 1989). An alternative form of this equation, which can be used to plot data, is

$$n \log c = -\log t + \text{constant}$$

(this constant is the logarithmic value of the constant in Equation 3). Although a wide range of values of n have been cited, usually the value appears to be close to 1 to 2. Where it is possible, the relationship should be derived from experimental data, ideally from a single series of experiments in the same laboratory and using the same strain of animal. If data are combined from different laboratories and different strains or species, the relationship generated may represent interlaboratory or interspecies (or interstrain) variation rather than a genuine concentration–time relationship.

Frequently there are insufficient data to verify the relationships and the value of n=1 is used. It is probably adequate when extrapolating to longer times, where it usually overestimates the consequences. However, the Haber rule could seriously underestimate if data are not available for short periods and extrapolation of information from longer exposure periods is undertaken. Because of underlying assumptions about 'steady-state' toxicokinetics inherent in any of these estimates at very short time intervals (say, less than 5 min) while equilibration to some form of pseudo steady states is taking place. Usually it is necessary to define the concentration-time combination for a boundary condition rather than for the mid-point value for an effect. Ideally this should be obtained from experimental data. Often it has to be derived from the slope of the dose-response curve. If data on the slope are not available, it may be possible to use an arbitrary ratio gleaned from generalized information available in the literature. Based on the comparison of the slightly weaker criterion 'evident toxicity' and LD_{50} for the same classification for oral toxicity in young healthy adults rats (where the ratio was 4-5 fold), the ratio for the relationship between 'dangerous dose' and LC_{50} could be about a threefold reduction in concentration in the same population.

A further reduction in concentration of 3-4 fold has been suggested for transfer from a general healthy population to population containing a high proportion of 'highly susceptible' people (see above). Thus, the slope of the dose-response curve depends on the type of population being studies. In transferring from LC_{50} or EC_x (representing the boundary death-disability), it is necessary to consider population heterogeneity. The total change from an LC_{50} for a recent study using young health adult inbred to the boundary death-disability for an outbred poorly healthy mixed age and strain population of rats could be an order of magnitude (tenfold) or more. A similar order of magnitude change has been proposed in moving from the criterion of death in a normal human population to 'dangerous dose' for a population containing a large number of 'highly susceptible' people (Health and Safety Executive, 1989a, see above).

As an alternative to the approach to concentration-time relationships outlined above, it is sometimes possible to describe mathematically a line for the boundary conditions of the concentration-time relationship using scatter diagrams, showing all concentrations and times at which the effect occurred (ECETOC, 1991). This approach normally requires access to more detailed data, including, ideally, the results for individual animals. It also can suffer from problems relating to population heterogeneity and interspecies and interlaboratory variation.

Additional Points

Whatever information emerges from animal toxicity data must always be compared with any data that are available for man. If there are no human data but data are available from several animal species, then those from the most sensitive species are normally chosen as representing a conservative approach unless there is good reason for considering that species anomalous.

□□□

Index

●●●